AF894399

C Y O'Connor ERADE Village Foundation

Education, Research and Development, Employment

Excerpt from a CYOEVF publication showing how similarities in animal genetics can help in the understanding of human disease

Interspecies Translation: Bovine Marbling to Human Muscular Dystrophy

By Jose L. Valenzuela, Sally S. Lloyd, Edward J. Steele, Francis l. Mastaglia and Roger L Dawkins

(In Muscular Dystrophies) Submitted: September 26th 2018
Reviewed: November 23rd 2018 Published: March 1st 2019

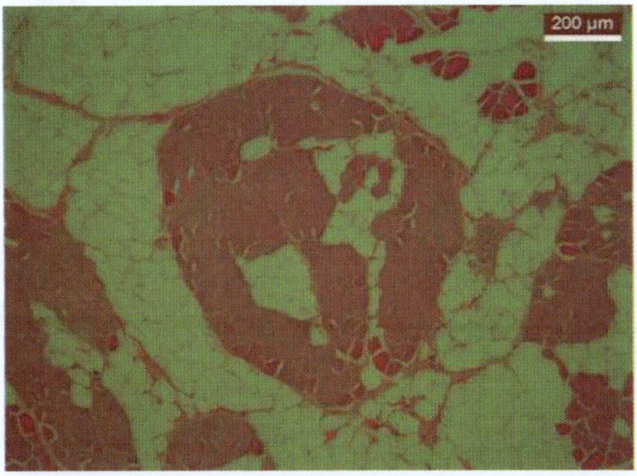

Figure 6: Histological section of Sacroaudalis dorsalis medialis of highly marbled, high Wagyu Content steer (88%) (wy63 ak25 dx13), showing aggressive adipose invasion, with abundant perimysial connective tissue and the generation of island-like areas of fibres with evident arch architectural changes including shrinkage of fibres as the front advances. Formalin-fixed H & E, MSA MB 1100, DOF 471, CYO lab number Ch18/110G.

36th Annual Report 2019

C Y O'Connor ERADE Village Foundation Inc

Street Address	24 Genomics Rise, Piara Waters WA 6112
	5 Del Park Road, North Dandalup WA 6207
Postal Address	PO Box 5100, Canning Vale South WA 6155
Telephone	(+61 8) 9397 1556

Key Contact	Professor Roger Dawkins
Email	rldawkins@cyo.edu.au
Second Contact	Dr Sally Lloyd
Email	slloyd@cyo.edu.au

Company Overview:

The C Y O'Connor Education Research and Development, Employment (ERADE) Village Foundation is a charitable foundation that conducts independent and sponsored research.

Product/Service Information:

To support inventors and researchers. Major aims are to understand evolution in the context of genomic prospecting and the development of diagnostic tests for inherited traits of medical and agricultural interest.

Published by Nearurban LLC,
8338 Puma Court
San Angelo, TX 76901
Tel (402) 310-1327
Email : admin@nearurban.net

Manufactured and printed by Kindle Direct

ISBN: 978-0-9864115-6-4

NU Publishing

Table of Contents

Board of Management

Executive Reports

Chairman's Report

Professor Roger Dawkins

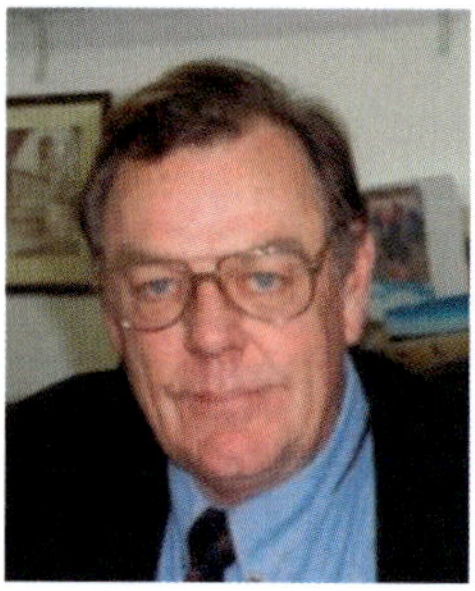

It is pleasing to have the opportunity to take a breath and provide updates on our many activities and to acknowledge those who are responsible for our success.

ON TRACK

North Dandalup CYOEVF Village

The renovation of "Ambrosa House" at 5 Del Park Road, has created a conference centre for seventy, a boardroom for twelve, a shared workspace for eight, four incubator offices and a self-contained apartment. We are now able to accept applications for start-ups.

We acknowledge our support foundation, Specific Diagnostics Pty Ltd ATF AL & M Dawkins Foundation (SDPL), which has invested approximately $1 million in the project and we are grateful to Capewest Investments Pty Ltd for efficient and painless execution, including renovation of the adjoining laboratory. Fortunately, this will be commissioned when the servicing can be extended. We will then have the opportunity to accommodate ten additional inventors since the Foundation continues to use the "Keilman Dairy" laboratory at 1574 Hopelands Road, Nambeelup

Earthworks and servicing of the Foundation's adjacent area of Lot 302, Southwest Highway and 7 Del Park Road, has been inspected and approved by the Shire of Murray. The total eligible expenditure to date is $1,876,193 (not including sand sourced from Mundup Farm). So far $153,994 of the 50% has been reimbursed by the Building Better Regions Fund (BBRF).

Problem Solving in Peel

Thanks in large measure to the grant from the WA Department of Jobs, Training, Science and Industry (JTSI), we have been able to respond to local requests as detailed in the report by Paul Fitzpatrick.

Kikuyu: For Improved Pasture and Nutrient Stripping

Thanks to support from the Peel Development Commission (PDC), we have defined new varieties that have adapted to local conditions. It is now possible to identify the components of mixed pastures with a view to improving silage and reducing unpleasant taints that limit the value of grass fed meat (see report by Tony Lloyd with submitted manuscript).

Better Barley for Peel

Our patented DNA test has identified markers for varieties and, more importantly, a potential method for identifying critical retrotransposons, which are responsible for adaptation to local environment and drive commercial value. We intend to test new varieties for their value as stockfeed, also as beer, given the ability to conduct trials of consumer preference in the licensed premises.

Livestock Genetics for Improved Meat Quality

We now have yet further evidence demonstrating the importance of the BOTA C19 haplotypes, such as 60.1, 60.7 and 30.4, in improving quality, value and consumer preference even when heterozygous in first crosses. See summary of Jose Valenzuela's PhD thesis.

On 27 September, 2019, Dr Daniel Hammond presented the data to the American Wagyu Association and came away with more than forty requests for testing.

Challenges

We see the need for an active training program so there are farmers, food handlers, technicians and analysts to cater for the expansion of the Peel Food Bowl. If so, research and development will be driven by demand rather than charitable funding.

Although the Foundation had to assume the full burden of funding the "BBRF" project and then retrospectively seeking reimbursements, the Board agreed to do so and has the funds available. This is in addition to the $1 million spent by SDPL but not considered relevant by BBRF. SDPL could provide a further $500,000 but this should not be necessary since the Foundation still has three buildings at Piara Waters that are expected to improve in value. I am not alone in wondering why there appear to be some confused messages arising from some of those competing for federal and state funding. Some of our plans have been replicated in Nambeelup giving the impression of unnecessary duplication. In fact, CYOEVF remains flexible and will be delighted if some of the necessary infrastructure can be available nearby, thereby freeing CYOEVF to focus on its core vision of multidisciplinary, independent, producer driven research and development.

We are grateful to Murdoch University for providing on-costs for staff and look forward to future one-on-one relationships. Subject to assurances, we wish to terminate the collaborative agreement in favour of a project-by-project relationship rather than PhD projects. We thank Professors David Morrison, Richard Harper and Li Chengdao for their encouragement. We will continue to inform them of international opportunities such as those now available through our local, national and international collaborations. However, the experience of the last three years indicates that CYOEVF must remain sufficiently independent to be able to respond to the needs of local farmers and their communities. We hope to support trainees and involve them in well-designed trials intended to have local benefits. Funding for such initiatives is a challenge but less so if the funds are controlled locally. This is one reason why we prefer project-by-project relationships with Murdoch University and with the CRC for Future Food Systems.

Acknowledgements

I thank the members and Board for their resolve in bringing our plans to this stage. We are grateful to the PDC and JTSI for financial support. I record my indebtedness to all Board members but single out Tony Lloyd, Alan Peggs, Renny Lee-Steere, Rob Giura, Jason Wallis, Ben Dawkins and Noel Jones who have taken specific responsibilities for new initiatives.

Also to non-Board members Sally Lloyd, Lindsay Baker and Paul Fitzpatrick. I simply observe that it is not easy to be multidisciplinary, independent and yet cohesive but, in my view, increasingly important that we remain so.

Postscript

BBRF

TMG remains committed to its contribution to the BBRF project which will ensure the relocation of T-Block and, subject to alternative advice, the residential accommodation. In the meanwhile, there have been complications in relation to Shire approvals. For example, the Shire has objected to its own Section 40 of December 2018, meaning that a tasting centre is no longer practical. Fortunately, TMG can now provide the same service at Byford as well as at CYO Pub. In addition, AL&MDF has almost completed the renovation of the Ambrosa Meeting Centre which can continue to provide an adequate hub plus accommodation. There is no immediate need for an additional meeting and tasting site. The food processing centre became an issue when we discovered that it does not accord with the BBRF specifications. Fortunately, there are now preferable alternatives which will not involve expenditure by the BBRF or the CYOEVF. Therefore, TMG has withdrawn its offer to fit-out, rent and manage the two buildings referred to as the "NDRC". These can be devoted to Incubators including the current five applicants.

The Building Projects Subcommittee of Jason Wallis, Tim Connoley, Aaron LoCicero and Rob Giura has engaged Brad Schrader of Realcom to manage the BBRF project and prepare the Incubators at Piara Waters for sale.

Murdoch University

Dr Sally Lloyd has transferred her employment to CYOEVF but retains an academic appointment with Murdoch University.

Shire of Murray (SOM)

CYOEVF has engaged Ed Turner to work with the Shire to define a plan for the North Dandalup CYOEVF Village with a primary focus on the immediate site provided by Goldfather.

This is now limited by planning restrictions. This project will be slow and incremental and should be driven largely by demands of Incubator tenants.

USA

License agreements have been developed and agreed. Our strategy is to move activities to collaborations where there is increasing demand, thanks largely to presentations by John Dawkins, Alan Peggs and Aaron Cooper.

Immediate Future

The Foundation has three commitments:

(a) Development of intellectual property through collaboration, as is happening in the US and Australia, particularly in the Peel region.

(b) Provision of facilities for multidisciplinary incubators and progression to start-ups. We recognise that success will be dependent on building a new community in which to "live, work and play".

(c) Support of Transform Peel and the Nambeelup Business Park, where compatible.

* * *

Vice-Chairman's Report — Mr Anthony Lloyd

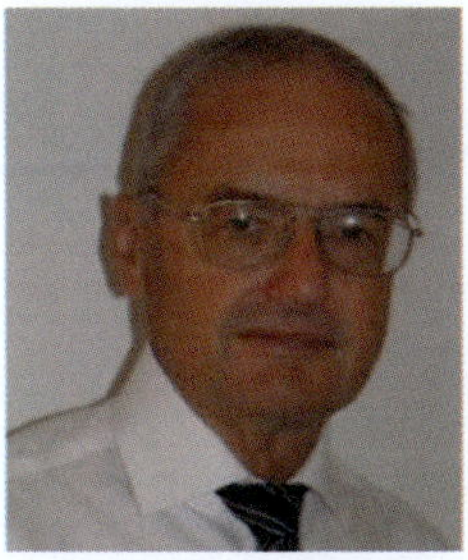

CONSTITUTION AND GOVERNANCE

Recent changes in the Associations Incorporation Act (WA) prompted a review of our constitution during the year.

In most respects the existing constitution complied with the updated requirements specified in the legislation. In addition to some technical matters, the constitution was amended in accordance with the Act to prohibit most payments to Board members without General Meeting approval. The existing policy of the Foundation is that Board members are not paid for services they provide to the Foundation, so no change to the Foundation's operations will result.

The opportunity was also taken to simplify the Foundation's name to "The C Y O'Connor ERADE Village Foundation Incorporated". The previous name included reference to the Foundation's origins in Immunology and molecular genetics research but which is no longer necessary to refer to in our name. The Foundation's constitution in other respects provides a flexible basis for carrying out its operations. It permits the borrowing of money (if necessary), leasing of land and the maintenance and management of the Foundation's Intellectual Property portfolio.

The Foundation has "Deductible Gift Recipient" status with the Australian Taxation Office, meaning that donors to the Foundation may reduce their taxable income by the amount or value of the gift. The ATO gave approval to the constitutional changes as not affecting our DGR status.

Recently the Board adopted a Conflict of Interest Policy based on the template published by the Australian Charities and Not-for-profits Commission, providing for Board members to record any relevant interest in a register maintained by CYOEVF.

Profiles

Deputy Research Director's Profile

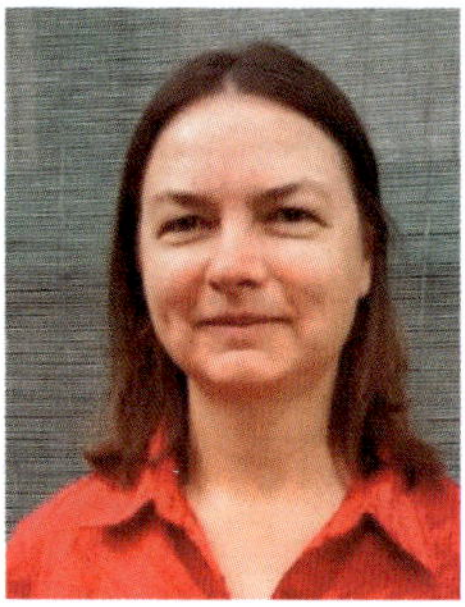

Dr Sally S Lloyd, BSc (Hons), PhD

Dr Lloyd studied physics at Murdoch University and graduated in 1993 with first class honours. Her research project within Alcoa's bauxite refinery was funded by a scholarship from the A J Parker Cooperative Research Centre for Hydrometallurgy. Alcoa later funded an extension of this work, employing Dr Lloyd as a Research Assistant into 2004.

In 1995, Dr Lloyd commenced her postdoctoral studies at the Australian National University (ANU) where she adapted a computer program, developed by Professor Takaya Hayashi of the National Institute of Fusion Science in Japan, to model plasma confinement and magnetic islands within the ANU's stellarator. A visit to Japan to further this collaboration included a trip to Mt Aso where she first saw Akaushi cattle – not, at the time, recognising their future importance. Dr Lloyd completed her PhD in Computational Plasma Physics in 2002. After graduating from ANU, Dr Lloyd moved to Townsville where she taught physics at James Cook University before running a diagnostic laboratory testing lubrication oil.

Since starting with the CYOEV Foundation as a Research Associate in 2012, Dr Lloyd has applied her physics knowledge to develop a test for the melting point of beef fat and in interpreting genetic information and primer design. Dr Lloyd became Deputy Research Director of the Foundation in 2015 and is responsible for the research team and for the supervision of Murdoch University postgraduate and other students and trainees. In addition, she chairs local research meetings and retreats and supervises diagnostic services for livestock paternity, provenance of food, pasture content and melting temperature of "healthy" intramuscular fat. Scientific publications, patents and presentations at national and international conferences attest to her productivity.

Friends of the CYOEVF

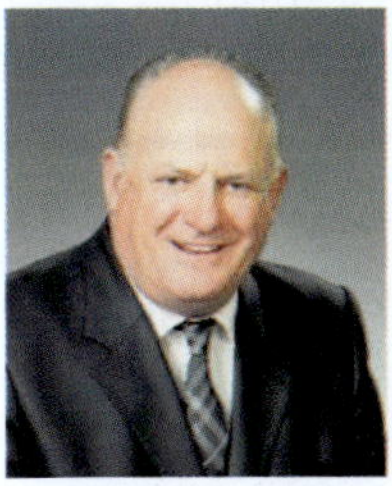

Mr Paul Fitzpatrick

The last twelve months has been an exciting and very positive period for the organisation and the people involved in our endeavours.

This has been my second year with the Foundation and the main focus has been on securing funding/partners for the development of the North Dandalup ERADE Village. The civil works at the Village are well under way. We have secured support via community involvement with the expert advisory committee that has been established with specialist people from the local community and individuals with agriculture expertise. This committee meets on a regular basis in conjunction with our weekly Wednesday lunch meetings.

We have also received positive support from the State Government for the Problem Solving in Peel (PSIP) program. This program is run through the department of Jobs, Tourism, Science and Innovation. We have secured support via community involvement with the expert advisory committee that has been established with specialist people from the local community and individuals with agriculture expertise. This committee met on a regular basis in conjunction with our weekly Wednesday lunch meetings. We have run a number of presentations on agriculture related issues at the Village where we discuss problems that are identified within the Peel region. In addition, we advise on proposed solutions to ensure better outcomes within the overall community. Some of the problems we have discussed and recommended solutions include:

- Toxic grasses
- Improved soils
- New industry
- Potential of solar power in irrigation and farming systems
- Agriculture applications of networked sensors and drone technology

- Sugar content test for silage making
- DNA testing for Pasture composition and
- Improved water supply for North Dandalup
- Farm Security

The success of this program has been outstanding and has allowed direct involvement by members of the farming and local community. Through this program we plan to announce our first participants for the Incubators and start-ups in the Village.

The announcement from Major General Michael Jeffery (Retired) who chairs the Soils for Life program relates to his visits to the Centre over the last twelve months. The Soils for Life program is an initiative that was established by the Australian government in 2012 with a strong focus on regenerative farming practices to ensure we have a healthy food zone, soil and water management for the region. It is proposed that North Dandalup will be one of two sites identified for trials in Western Australia.

We commit to irrigation avenues as a new strategy which encompasses regenerative sustainable agriculture, rotational grazing and silage production, worm and dung beetle management, land and tree care, nutrient stripping, best welfare practice, opportunities for pasture trials, improved biosecurity and infection control, daily inspection, renewable energy, efficient fertigation, etc.

The *Friends of the CY O'Connor ERADE Village Foundation* intention is to encourage community involvement in the activities of the Foundation. Specifically:

- Support of researchers and inventors.
- Events, such as the charity golf day, charity auctions of donated art, invitations to distinguished visitors.
- Improvements to the North Dandalup Village.

* * *

Financial Statements

IMMUNOGENETICS RESEARCH FOUNDATION WA INC
T/A
THE C.Y. O'CONNOR ERADE VILLAGE FOUNDATION
ABN: 67 161 830 965

CONTENTS

Auditors Independence Declaration

Under Section 307C of the Corporations Act 2001

To Members of the CY O'Connor Erade Village Foundation

I declare that, to the best of my knowledge and belief, in relation to the audit of the CY O'Connor Erade Village Foundation for the year ended 31 December 2018 there have been:

(a) No contraventions to the auditor independence requirement of the Corporations Act 2001 in relation to the audit; and

(b) No contraventions of any applicable code of professional conduct in relation to the audit.

John Pascoe (FCPA)
Registered Company Audit No. 13479

Dated this 2nd April 2019

IMMUNOGENETICS RESEARCH FOUNDATION WA INC
T/A
THE C.Y. O'CONNOR ERADE VILLAGE FOUNDATION
ABN: 67 161 830 965
C Y O'CONNOR HI-TECH INCUBATOR CENTRE
DEPARTMENTAL TRADING, PROFIT AND LOSS STATEMENT
FOR THE YEAR ENDED 31 DECEMBER 2018

	Note	2018 $	2018 $
C Y O'CONNOR HI-TECH INCUBATOR CENTRE			
OTHER INCOME			
Lease Rentals		230,516	217,480
EXPENSES			
Bad Debts Written Off	2	818	-
Cleaning		-	4,160
Depreciation - Plant & Equipment	3	1,633	2,003
Depreciation - Buildings		25,151	25,886
Electricity		-	9,653
Leasing Fees		12,720	9,561
Incubator Management Fees		16,383	6,787
Repairs & Maintenance	4	3,203	14,608
		59,908	72,658
SURPLUS (DEFICIT) FROM INCOME AND EXPENDITURE		170,608	144,822
Opening Balance 1st January 2018		1,625,937	1,481,115
Closing Balance 31st December 2018		1,796,545	1,625,937

IMMUNOGENETICS RESEARCH FOUNDATION WA INC
T/A
THE C.Y. O'CONNOR ERADE VILLAGE FOUNDATION
ABN: 67 161 830 965
RESEARCH & GENERAL FUND
DEPARTMENTAL TRADING, PROFIT AND LOSS STATEMENT
FOR THE YEAR ENDED 31 DECEMBER 2018

	Note	2018 $	2017 $
RESEARCH & GENERAL			
Donations / Bequests		155,188	37,918
Fund Raising		5,296	7,279
Meeting Registration Fees		3,990	3,290
Membership Fees		3,227	6,818
Laundry & Gaming Machine Sales		2,570	730
		170,271	56,035
OTHER INCOME			
Grant Income		125,000	55,000
Interest Received		34,014	31,707
SubLease Rentals		1,620	-
Other Income		-	1
Reimbursements & Recoups		-	1,696
Capital Gain / (Loss) on Sale of Non-Current Assets		(9,792)	-
Profit / (Loss) on Sale of Non-current Assets		884	-
		151,726	88,404
EXPENSES			
Accountancy & Audit Fees		5,860	5,482
Advertising		248	160
Bank Charges		95	235
Bad Debts Written Off	2	491	-
Cleaning		1,468	1,561
Consultancy Fees		78,450	14,838
Contract Work		266,177	995
Computer Expense		3,420	-
Depreciation - Plant & Equipment	3	17,637	19,356
Electricity		-	177
Fees & Permits		284	8,080
Freight & Cartage		743	1,903
Fund Raising Costs		-	1,000
Fuel & Oil		119	-
Gas		390	-
Insurance		15,927	10,326
Interest Paid		31	3
Legal Cost		300	-
Licensing Fees		1,628	763
Meeting / Visitors / Honorarium		25,204	18,031
Consumables & Lab Supplies		23,737	36,366
Motor Vehicle Expense		100	-
Patent Fees		1,360	27,153

IMMUNOGENETICS RESEARCH FOUNDATION WA INC
T/A
THE C.Y. O'CONNOR ERADE VILLAGE FOUNDATION
ABN: 67 161 830 965
RESEARCH & GENERAL FUND
DEPARTMENTAL TRADING, INCOME AND EXPENDITURE
FOR THE YEAR ENDED 31 DECEMBER 2018

	Note	2018 $	2017 $
Postage		630	717
Printing & Stationery		4,760	532
Rent - 5 Del Park Road		90,000	-
Repairs & Maintenance	4	11,425	482
Research & Development Costs		84	-
Scholarships		39,847	-
Subscriptions		314	1,325
Superannuation Contributions		650	7,921
Travelling Expenses		296	-
Uniforms		586	-
Unrealised Loss / (Gain) on Shares		-	(24,033)
Wages		8,470	83,753
Waste Disposal		1,096	438
Water		168	-
		601,995	217,564
SURPLUS (DEFICIT) FROM INCOME AND EXPENDITURE		(279,998)	(73,125)
Opening Balance 1st January 2018		1,040,852	1,113,977
Closing Balance 31st December 2018		760,854	1,040,852

IMMUNOGENETICS RESEARCH FOUNDATION WA INC
T/A
THE C.Y. O'CONNOR ERADE VILLAGE FOUNDATION
ABN: 67 161 830 965
BALANCE SHEET
AS AT 31 DECEMBER 2018

	Note	2018 $	2017 $
TRUST FUNDS			
RESERVES	5	2,557,399	2,666,789
TOTAL TRUST FUNDS		2,557,399	2,666,789
Represented by:			
CURRENT ASSETS			
Cash on Hand		1	1
Petty Cash		108	113
Prepayments on Contract		-	42,282
Westpac Max 112867		34,028	7,204
Westpac Research Account 10-4752		121,071	7,207
Westpac Community Solutions Account 1645		23,680	3,870
Westpac Community Solution 2961		1,087	3,000
Term Deposits	6	1,300,314	1,308,020
Accounts Receivable		27,635	3,575
Loans - Unsecured	7	10,000	10,000
GST Refundable (Payable)		13,915	(2,885)
TOTAL CURRENT ASSETS		1,531,839	1,382,387
NON CURRENT ASSETS			
Fixed Assets			
5 Del Park Road Reserch Facility - Capitalised Expenses		26,556	-
Computer Equipment		364,971	364,971
Less: Accumulated Depreciation		(364,542)	(364,273)
		429	698
Motor Vehicles		-	13,500
Less: Accumulated Depreciation		-	(12,943)
		-	557
Office Furniture & Equipment		11,612	11,612
Less: Accumulated Depreciation		(11,269)	(11,183)
		343	429
Laboratory Equipment		561,092	561,092
Less: Accumulated Depreciation		(476,830)	(459,625)
		84,262	101,467
Incubators		55,124	55,124
Less: Accumulated Depreciation		(47,190)	(45,557)
		7,934	9,567
Incubator Buildings		1,287,625	1,287,625
Less: Accumulated Depreciation		(338,448)	(313,297)
		949,177	974,328
Total Fixed Assets		1,068,701	1,087,046

IMMUNOGENETICS RESEARCH FOUNDATION WA INC
T/A
THE C.Y. O'CONNOR ERADE VILLAGE FOUNDATION
ABN: 67 161 830 965
BALANCE SHEET
AS AT 31 DECEMBER 2018

	Note	2018 $	2017 $
Investments			
Listed Shares in Public Companies	8	-	156,217
Patents		88,860	54,750
Total Investments		88,860	210,967
TOTAL NON CURRENT ASSETS		1,157,561	1,298,013
TOTAL ASSETS		2,689,400	2,680,400
CURRENT LIABILITIES			
Trade Creditors		123,356	3,768
Incubator Bond Monies	9	5,020	7,970
Amounts Withheld	10	3,625	1,873
TOTAL CURRENT LIABILITIES		132,001	13,611
TOTAL LIABILITIES		132,001	13,611
NET ASSETS		2,557,399	2,666,789

IMMUNOGENETICS RESEARCH FOUNDATION WA INC
T/A
THE C.Y. O'CONNOR ERADE VILLAGE FOUNDATION
ABN: 67 161 830 965
NOTES TO THE FINANCIAL STATEMENTS
FOR THE YEAR ENDED 31 DECEMBER 2018

	2018	2017
	$	$

1 Statement of Significant Accounting Policies

The director of the trustee company has prepared the financial statements of the trust on the basis that the trust is a non-reporting entity because there are no users dependent on general purpose financial statements. The financial statements are therefore special purpose financial statements that have been prepared in order to meet the needs of beneficiaries.

The financial statements have been prepared in accordance with the significant accounting policies disclosed below which the director has determined are appropriate to meet the needs of members. Such accounting policies are consistent with the previous period unless stated otherwise.

The financial statements have been prepared on an accruals basis and are based on historical costs unless otherwise stated in the notes. The accounting policies that have been adopted in the preparation of these statements are as follows:

Property, Plant and Equipment

Property, plant and equipment are carried at cost, independent or director's valuation. All assets, excluding freehold land and buildings are depreciated over the useful lives of the assets to the trust.

Increases in the carrying amount arising on revaluation of land and buildings are credited to a revaluation reserve in shareholders' equity. Decreases that offset previous increases of the same asset are charged against fair value reserves directly in equity; all other decreases are charged to the income statement. Each year the difference between depreciation based on the revalued carrying amount of the asset charged to the income statement and depreciation based on the asset's original cost is transferred from the revaluation reserve to retained earnings.

The carrying amount of plant and equipment is reviewed annually by directors to ensure it is not in excess of the recoverable amount from these assets. The recoverable amount is assessed on the basis of the expected net cash flows that will be received from the asset's employment and subsequent disposal. The expected net cash flows have not been discounted in determining recoverable amounts.

Property, Plant and Equipment (PPE)

Leasehold improvements and office equipment are carried at cost less, where applicable, any accumulated depreciation.

The depreciable amount of all PPE is depreciated over the useful lives of the assets to the trust commencing from the time the asset is held ready for use.

Leasehold improvements are amortised over the shorter of either the unexpired period of the lease or the estimated useful lives of the improvements.

IMMUNOGENETICS RESEARCH FOUNDATION WA INC
T/A
THE C.Y. O'CONNOR ERADE VILLAGE FOUNDATION
ABN: 67 161 830 965
NOTES TO THE FINANCIAL STATEMENTS
FOR THE YEAR ENDED 31 DECEMBER 2018

		2018 $	2017 $
2	**Bad Debt Written Off**		
	Hi-Tech Incubator Centre	818	-
	Research & General Fund	491	-
		1,309	-
3	**Depreciation - Plant & Equipment**		
	Hi-Tech Incubator Centre	1,633	2,003
	Research & General Fund	17,637	19,356
		19,270	21,359
4	**Repairs & Maintenance**		
	Hi-Tech Incubator Centre	3,203	14,608
	Research & General Fund	11,425	482
		14,628	15,090
5	**RESERVES**		
	Reserves - Deficit	-	-
	7th MHC Evolution Meeting Fund	-	-
	C Y O'Connor Hi-Tech Incubator Centre	1,796,545	1,625,937
	Research & General Fund	760,854	1,040,852
		2,557,399	2,666,789
6	**Term Deposits**		
	Westpac Term Deposit 17-7599	105,268	102,650
	Westpac Term Deposit 18-6946	67,191	65,539
	Westpac Term Deposit 21-4134	100,000	131,913
	Westpac Term Deposit 21-4126	105,596	103,000
	Westpac Term Deposit 21-5671	131,594	128,384
	Westpac Term Deposit 21-9453	165,267	102,669
	Westpac Term Deposit 23-4151	106,864	104,176
	Westpac Term Deposit 23-4178	100,000	131,791
	Westpac Term Deposit 23-4186	107,376	104,706
	Westpac Term Deposit 21-1689	52,520	100,000
	Westpac Term Deposit 24-4819	104,890	102,331
	Westpac Term Deposit 24-9548	53,403	100,861
	Westpac Term Deposit 26-5932	-	30,000
	Westpac Term Deposit 26-5933	100,345	-
		1,300,314	1,308,020

IMMUNOGENETICS RESEARCH FOUNDATION WA INC
T/A
THE C.Y. O'CONNOR ERADE VILLAGE FOUNDATION
ABN: 67 161 830 965
NOTES TO THE FINANCIAL STATEMENTS
FOR THE YEAR ENDED 31 DECEMBER 2018

		2018 $	2017 $
7	**Loans - Unsecured**		
	E J Steele	10,000	10,000
		10,000	10,000
8	**Listed Shares in Public Companies**		
	Listed Shares in Public Companies at Market Value	-	156,216
9	**Incubator Bond Monies**		
	Auslanka	1,020	1,120
	Better Care Medical Centre	-	1,360
	Youme Clothing	-	450
	Spicy Wok	1,200	1,200
	Make Your Mark Art Cafe	-	1,040
	Renov8withus Pty Ltd	-	1,400
	Indebiti Solutions Pty Ltd	1,400	1,400
	Shearer Consulting	1,400	-
		5,020	7,970
10	**Amounts Withheld**		
	Amounts Withheld from Salary, Wages and Other Payments	1,102	-
	Employee Superannuation Payable	2,523	1,873
		3,625	1,873

Compilation Report

COMPILATION REPORT
IMMUNOGENETICS RESEARCH FOUNDATION WA INC
T/A
THE C.Y. O'CONNOR ERADE VILLAGE FOUNDATION
ABN: 67 161 830 965

We have compiled the accompanying special purpose financial statements of THE C.Y. O'CONNOR ERADE VILLAGE FOUNDATION which comprise the balance sheet as at 31 December 2018, profit and loss statement and cash flow statement for the year then ended, a summary of significant accounting policies and other explanatory notes.

The specific purpose for which these special purpose financial statements have been prepared is to provide information relating to the performance and financial position of the incorporated body that satisfies the information needs of the director

The responsibility of the Director

The director is solely responsible for the information contained in the special purpose financial statements and has determined that the basis of accounting used is appropriate to meet their needs and for the purpose for which the financial statements were prepared.

Our responsibility

On the basis of information provided by the director, we have compiled the accompanying special purpose financial statements in accordance with the financial reporting framework described in Note 1 to the financial statements and APES 315: Compilation of Financial Information.

Our procedures use accounting expertise to collect, classify and summarise the financial information, which the director provided, into a financial report. Our procedures do not include verification or validation procedures. No audit or review has been performed and accordingly no assurance is expressed.

The special purpose financial statements were prepared exclusively for the director. We do not accept responsibility to any other person for the content of the special purpose financial statements.

Name of Firm: Pascoe Partners Accountants

Name of Director: Wayne Michael Cox
MTax, Dip FS(FP), CPA, CTA

Address: Level 2, 100 Havelock Street West Perth

Dated: 28.3.19

Auditor's Report

JOHN D PASCOE, FCPA

Certified Practising Accountant
Registered Tax Agent
Registered Company Auditor

Unit 487
118 Monash Avenue
Nedlands
Western Australia 6010

ABN 64 724 120 246
Email: johnjill@westnet.com.au
Mob: 0406 380 215

2 April 2019

Chairperson
CY O'Connor Erade Foundation
Level 2/100 Havelock Street
WEST PERTH 6005

Dear Chairperson

INDEPENDENT AUDITOR'S REPORT

I have audited the accompanying financial report, being a special purpose financial report of The CY O'Connor Erade Village Foundation (association), which comprises the committee's report, the assets and liabilities statement as at 31 December 2018, the income and expenditure statement for the year ended on, notes comprising a summary of significant accounting policies and other explanatory information and the statement by members of the committee.

Committee's Responsibility for the Financial Report

The committee of The CY O'Connor Erade Village Foundation is responsible for preparation of the financial report, and has determined that the basis of preparation described in Note 1 is appropriate to meet the requirements of the Associations Incorporation Act (1987) and is appropriate to meet the needs of the members. The committee's responsibility also includes such internal control as the committee determines necessary to enable preparation of the financial report that is free from material misstatement, whether due to fraud or error.

Auditor's Responsibility

My responsibility is to express a conclusion on the financial report based on my audit. I conducted my audit in accordance with Auditing Standards. Those standards require that we comply with relevant ethical requirements relating to audit engagements and plan and perform the audit to obtain reasonable assurance whether the financial report is free from material misstatement

An audit involves performing procedures to obtain audit evidence about the amounts and disclosures in the financial report. The procedures selected depend on the auditor's judgement, including the assessment o f the risks of material misstatement of the financial report, whether due to fraud or error. In making those risk assessments, the auditor considers internal control relevant to the association's preparation of the financial report that gives a true and fair view, in order to design audit procedures that are appropriate in the circumstances, but not for the purpose of expressing an opinion on the effectiveness of the association's internal control. An Audit also includes evaluating the appropriateness of accounting policies used and the reasonableness of accounting estimates made by the committee, as well as evaluating the overall presentation of the financial report.

I believe that the audit evidence I have obtained is sufficient and appropriate to provide a basis for the audit opinion.

Qualification

In common with most charitable institutions receiving cash donations, the entity has determined that it is impractical to establish controls over cash donations before they are banked and recorded in the accounting system. As a result my audit was restricted to the amounts recorded in the accounting system.

Opinion

In my opinion, except for the effects on the financial report, if any that the above qualification may have on the financial report of The CY O'Connor Erade Village Foundation, the report presents fairly, in all material respects, the financial position of The CY O'Connor Erade Village Foundation as at 31 December 2018 and its financial performance for the year then ended in accordance with the accounting policies described in Note 1 to the financial statements, and the Associations Incorporation Act (1987).

Basis of Accounting and Restriction on Distribution

Without modifying my opinion, attention is drawn to Note 1 to the financial report, which describes the basis of accounting. The financial report has been prepared to assist The CY O'Connor Erade Village Foundation to meet the requirements of the Associations Incorporation Act (1987). As a result, the financial report may not be suitable for another purpose.

Should you have any queries on the above matter, please do not hesitate to contact me.

Kind regards

John Pascoe (FCPA)
Registered Company Audit No. 13479

Recent Publications

MHC Genomics and Disease: Looking Back to Go Forward

Roger L. Dawkins * and Sally S. Lloyd

Centre for Innovation in Agriculture, Murdoch University and C Y O'Connor ERADE Village Foundation, North Dandalup 6207, Western Australia. *Correspondence: rldawkins@cyo.edu.au
cells *Received: 14 June 2019; Accepted: 16 August 2019; Published: date 21 August 2019*

Abstract: Ancestral haplotypes are conserved but extremely polymorphic kilobase sequences, which have been faithfully inherited over at least hundreds of generations in spite of migration and admixture. They carry susceptibility and resistance to diverse diseases, including deficiencies of CYP21 hydroxylase (47.1) and complement components (18.1), as well as numerous autoimmune diseases (8.1). The haplotypes are detected by segregation within ethnic groups rather than by SNPs and GWAS. Susceptibility to some other diseases is carried by specific alleles shared by multiple ancestral haplotypes, e.g., ankylosing spondylitis and narcolepsy. The difference between these two types of association may explain the disappointment with many GWAS. Here we propose a pathway for combining the two different approaches. SNP typing is most useful after the conserved ancestral haplotypes have been defined by other methods.

Keywords: *MHC; ancestral haplotype; autoimmune disease*

1. Introduction

It has been very nearly 50 years since Terasaki, Brewerton, and their colleagues discovered the extraordinary association between ankylosing spondylitis (AS) and HLA B27 [1,2]. With a few caveats of great interest to clinicians, all patients with AS have this allele, justifying the idea that B27 is an essential requirement for the disease–effectively a sine qua non [3]. However, the allele is much more frequent than the disease, and is therefore not itself sufficient. Penetrance is low [4,5]. Other known requirements are male sex and adult age, indicating that the mechanisms of susceptibility and pathogenesis may be quite complex and difficult to unravel. This is still the case today, although the fundamental finding has been confirmed to exhaustion [6].

It has been nearly 40 years since it was established that other HLA associations are completely different [3,7]. For example, in Caucasoids, the more severe forms of systemic lupus erythematosus (SLE) and myasthenia gravis with thymic hyperplasia (MG) are associated with the 8.1 ancestral haplotype [8,9]. This sequence includes B8, but extends over more than a megabase from HLA A to HLA DP. The genetic factors responsible for susceptibility and severity must be numerous and widely spaced throughout the MHC, although most evidence implicates the central MHC, including the *C2*, *Bf*, *C4*, *HSP*, and *TNF* genes, together with their associated non-coding or regulatory sequences. In contrast to AS, female sex is important for these conditions. [10].

By 1983, these two different types of association were well recognized [8]. Over subsequent decades, many more examples have been added. Narcolepsy is another example of the allelic form in that the DQB1 0602 association is not restricted to one ethnic group [11,12]. Therefore, explanations for a direct role of a single allele are sought, in this case, and may ultimately appear to be disarmingly simple as for haemochromatosis [13,14] and some drug hypersensitivities [15].

Deficiencies of C4, C2, and 21-hydroxylase (21OH) are examples of associations with extensive ancestral haplotypes (8.1, 18.1, and 47.1, respectively) [16,17]. In each case, there is a plausible explanation, in that the particular sequence includes a missing or defective gene. The observations by Alper et al. [7,18,19] were important in leading to concepts of conserved population haplotypes, which have been faithfully inherited over thousands of generations and are best illustrated by 57.1, which is represented to various degrees in multiple ethnicities.

As different ancestral groups formed and migrated out of Africa and beyond, they carried conserved MHC sequences, which were fixed at each of the alpha, beta, gamma, and delta polymorphic frozen blocks (PFB) (see Figure 1 and Table 1).

These sequences were shuffled laterally somewhat as populations mixed, and new combinations appeared, but the more polymorphic regions survive to this day [20–22]. In the case of these deficiencies, the defective or missing *C4*, *C2*, or 21OH genes remain within the frozen sequence.

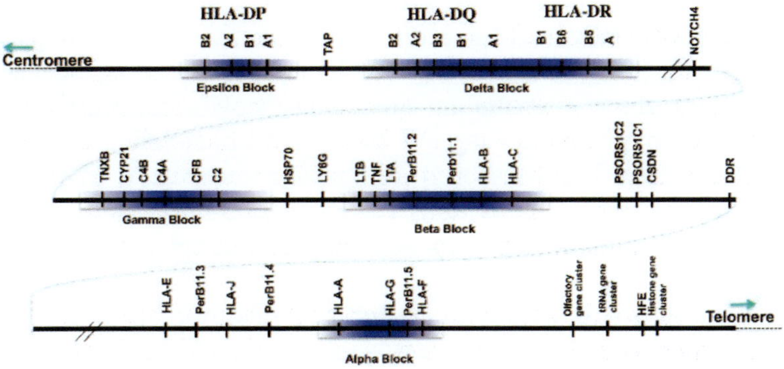

Figure 1. Polymorphic frozen blocks (PFB) in the MHC. Reproduced with permission from [5], and adapted from [16].

The organization of the MHC provides a model for the genome. Each ancestral haplotype has its own map. Polymorphic frozen blocks are shaded. Not all genes are shown. PerB11 is now designated *MIC*. Frozen refers to the freezing of the sequence by inhibition of recombination and mutations, whether

1. unequal crossing-over,
2. double recombination,
3. nucleotide replacement,
4. insertions and deletions,
5. duplication,
6. other.

It was only through extensive family studies that it became clear that recombination occurred outside polymorphic frozen blocks (Figure 2). Indeed, the frozen blocks must have been inherited faithfully over many generations, since identical haplotypes occur in subjects with extensive family trees showing no known relationship, and even in populations that were widely scattered geographically, implying only very remote common ancestry.

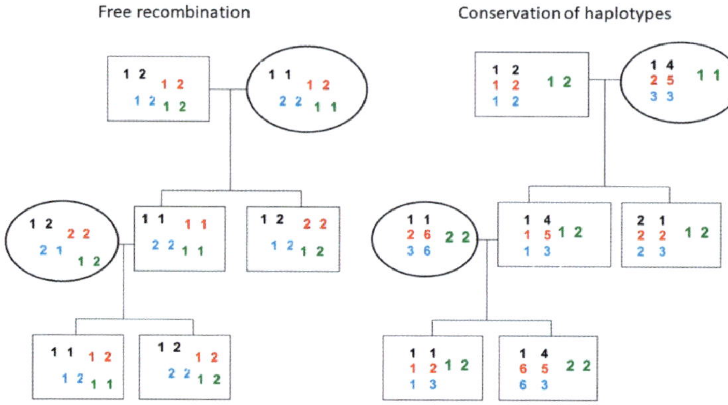

Figure 2. Stable segregation of ancestral haplotypes through three generation family trees. The left describes the inheritance pattern, where the loci are bi-allelic and segregate independently. The right describes the inheritance pattern within PFB, where the alleles are highly polymorphic and the four ancestral haplotypes have segregated predictably.

The reality is that the frozen blocks occupy only a limited proportion of the whole MHC region of a megabase or more, and we have not been able, as suggested in Figure 1, to define hard boundaries between frozen blocks and areas subject to recombination. This difficulty leads us to conclude that there are degrees of freezing as well as specific hotspots. Carrington [23] has contributed by identifying some of the regions which do recombine, but we suspect that such regions are dependent on the genomic environment rather than distance. For example, B8, which is Caucasoid specific by any measure, occurs in non- caucasoids with MG but hardly otherwise [24]. This observation implies that lateral transfer between haplotypes of very different ancestry may lead to thawing as a consequence of differences in the cis, trans, and epistatic interactions. Using multiethnic mapping is powerful [25–27] as a way to find which components carry susceptibility. In other words, ancestral haplotypes are preserved in ethnicities, but eventually fall apart in multiracial combinations.

Susceptibility to autoimmune diseases, such SLE, MG, and insulin-dependent diabetes mellitus (IDDM) must be similarly frozen [8,28–32]—although, to date, there is no mechanistic explanation for the susceptibility [20,32]. Largely, for this reason, we have suggested a dominant role for non-coding regulatory sequences associated with duplicons, indels, and retroviral-like elements (Table 1). We also implicate *epistatic, trans*, and *cis* interactions, with their potential to increase the degree of functional polymorphism exponentially [5,16]. *Epistatic* refers to sequences on different chromosomes, which segregate independently. *Trans* refers to the sequence of the second alternative chromosome. *Cis* refers to the same chromosome.

Table 1. Lessons from MHC genomics.

- Human diversity is inherited from ancestors, rather than created by recent mutation.
- Diversity is regenerated at speciation and maintained by meiotic recombination between the ancestral haplotypes within polymorphic frozen blocks.
- The unit of inheritance is the ancestral haplotype.
- Such sequences carry specific alleles, duplicons, indels and retroviral-like elements (RLEs), which together regulate gene expression.

Reproduced with permission from [5].

These lessons could not have been predicted from the prevailing concepts, which still underlie the thinking behind SNPs and GWAS (Table 2). This SNP-based thinking promotes an overemphasis on the role of ongoing mutation, compared to conservation of ancient polymorphism[33].

Table 2. Alternative dogma.

- Genetic diversity or inherited variation requires ongoing mutation.
- Diversity accumulates through errors in the copying of DNA.
- The unit of inheritance is the allele.
- At each locus alleles may be deleterious, beneficial, or neutral.
- Meiotic recombination scrambles maternal and paternal alleles.
- Linkage disequilibrium between SNPs defines haplotypes.

Reproduced with permission from [5].

Clearly, any understanding of MHC genomics leading to disease must take account of the pragmatic observations implicating age- and sex-dependent penetrance. In Figure 3, we illustrate the potential importance of cis and trans interactions by proposing that ancestral haplotypes can be represented by meshing polymorphic cogs. The degree of meshing or interaction, whether cis or trans, is affected by size and density (expression), as well as by competition with similar cogs, including those representing paralogous sequences encoded on other chromosomes. Thus, MHC, genotypically identical subjects may be affected to different degrees (Figure 3).

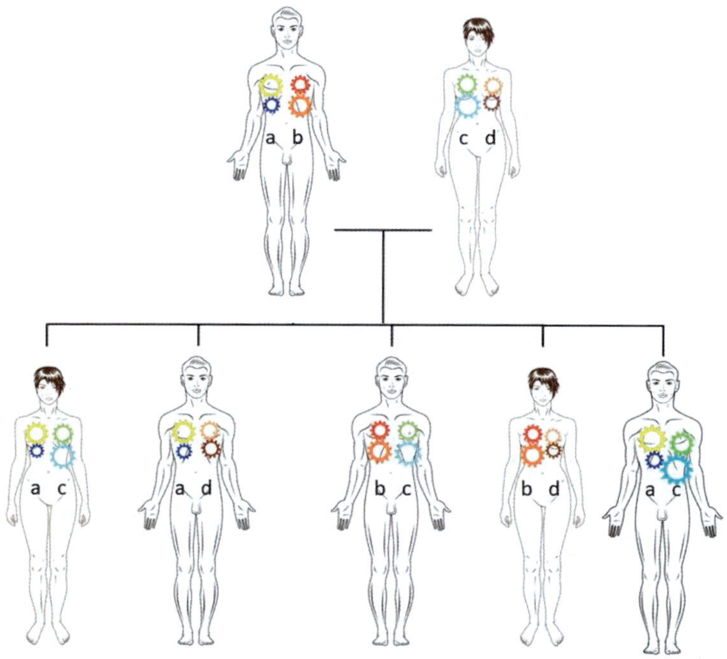

Figure 3. Segregating ancestral haplotypes preserve cis interactions. Ancestral haplotypes are represented by two cogs meshing vertically (in *cis*). The size and shape of cogs represent polymorphism or variant forms of the blocks. For example, the father has yellow–blue (**a**) and red–orange (**b**) haplotypes while the mother has green-cyan (c) and orange-brown (d) haplotypes. Haplotype (**a**) has been transmitted to the eldest daughter, eldest son, and youngest son. The middle two children have inherited haplotype (**b**). Reactive meshing is dependent on hormonal and other environmental influences. The oldest and youngest offspring are genotypically identical, but the interactions are different as a consequence of the sexual environment. Adapted with permission from [5].

These models have led to the concept of multifunctional polymorphic control of metabolic and other pathways. Cascades involving stepwise activation of related products, such as the complement system, are promising targets for further study.

2. Recognition of Conserved Ancestral Haplotypes

Table 3 illustrates how ancestral haplotypes were recognized initially. Today there are many more haplotypic markers, including noncoding sequences between the loci shown. As the number of haplotypic markers increased, including SNPs, it became more and more obvious that very few are haplo-specific. It follows that linkage disequilibrium (LD) cannot define such haplotypes. For example, 2 × 2 delta values cannot identify 18.1 and 18.2, because the alleles are shared by other haplotypes.

Table 3. Haplotype definitions and frequencies in an Australian population.

Ancestral Haplotype	A	Cw	B	C2	Bf	C4A	C4B	DR	DQ	Frequency
7.1	3	7	7	C	S	3	1	2	6	12.9%
8.1	1	7	8	C	S	0	1	3	2	13.2%
13.1			13		S	3	1	7		2.6%
18.1	25	-	18	0	S	4	2	3	6	1.1%
18.2	30	5	18	C	F1	3	0	3	2	1.7%
18.3			18		S	3	1	5		5.2%
35.1		4	35		S	3	1	5		6.9%
35.2	3	4	35	C	F	3 + 2	0	1	5	0.9%
35.3	11	4	35		S	3	0	1	5	2.3%
44.1	2	5	44	C	S	3	0	4	7	5.5%
44.2	29	4	44	C	F	3	1	7	2	2.6%
47.1	3	6	47	C	F	1	0	7	2	<0.6%
57.1	1	6	57	C	S	6	1	7	9	2.6%
65.1		8	65	C	S	2	1 + 2	1	5	0.6%

Adapted from [34] and [35].

3. Genome-Wide Association Studies and Single Nucleotide Polymorphisms

We believe that the above concepts and models of ancestral haplotypes suggest an alternative approach to the conduct and analysis for genome-wide association studies. When applied to the MHC, some results of commercial SNP typing have been disappointing, even to the point that a recent review by Kennedy et al. [36] essentially dismisses the many classic studies, and very unwisely blames "HLA typing errors, disregard of population structure and lack of replication" [36]. The same authors cite a paper which promotes a "focus on haplotypes …

first suggested in 1987", thereby ignoring important previous contributions on haplotypes—including the original use of the term in 1967 by Ruggero Ceppellini [37,38]—and a huge body of careful observations that have been confirmed repeatedly and rediscovered, without attribution, in the past few decades.
The International Hapmap Project [39–41] is a potentially valuable resource of high-resolution SNP-typed individuals, and includes samples of cell lines used to define the genomic sequence of conserved, extended ancestral haplotypes, which segregate faithfully through families. Surprisingly, the proponents and users [42] of Hapmap have ignored the opportunities for reconciliation with earlier studies, which addressed the shortcomings of LD analysis and focused on haplotypic sequences, including RLEs; indels; duplications; and single nucleotide polymorphism in the literal sense, used by Gaudieri et al. [43] and Longman et al. [44] to map regions of extensive, interrupted sequence differences. The importance of PFB [16] or fixity [45] was also ignored until rediscovered [46].
A more balanced review by Petersdorf and O'hUigin [47] begins the daunting process of integrating population genetics, classic HLA associations, ancestral haplotypes, polymorphic frozen blocks, SNP typing, and gene expression [47]. The authors hope for "the study of haplotype-associated phenotypic differences" and for "haplotype-matching" in transplantation. Indeed, there is already great encouragement for each of these ambitions. The functional differences conferred by ancestral haplotypes, such as 8.1, have been well known for more than 30 years, and include *TNF* and *IgA* concentrations, even though the latter is not encoded within the MHC [16,48,49]. The benefit of haplotype matching in renal and bone marrow transplantation was established decades ago [50,51].

4. Reconciling MHC Genomics and SNP Typing

While we recognize that the disconnect between classical MHC and later SNP genomics will decrease [47,52], we hope this happens quickly. To this end, we summarize the issues as follows:

1. There is no possibility of a single reference sequence. Rather, there are numerous ancestral haplotypes, each with its own very extensive and specific sequence [35,53–55].

2. These sequences are characteristic of ancestral populations or ethnicities. SNP typing on heterozygous mixed populations cannot reveal ancestral haplotype—or at least, must be extremely inefficient [20].
3. MHC complexity is best managed by defining haplotypes through segregation in extensive family studies [56]—not trios—since the power of segregation increases with the number of copies in different heterozygous combinations. Recombination can be demonstrated given sufficient generations to study.
4. Ancestral haplotypes include specific duplications, indels, etc. [54]. Fortunately, there are now many panels of homozygous cell lines and libraries of their sequences available [57,58]. These should be the references and should replace allele and SNP databases.
5. Penetrance is crucial but complex, and depends on age, sex, and a multitude of environmental factors that will vary from time to time and in different settings [53]. Cis and trans interactions are well known contributors to susceptibility and severity [5] These need to be included in the experimental design, but will be difficult to understand until the relevant pathways are defined. We recommend careful consideration of the concept of whole genome duplications resulting in paralogous sequences [16,59], which may compete with and modify the effect of any sequence implicated through SNP analysis.
6. Linkage disequilibrium (LD) is an incomplete reflection of conserved haplotypes and their relative frequencies. Many highly conserved haplotypes cannot be detected by delta values, because even though haplotypic (i.e., present on all examples), individual SNPs are *not* haplo-specific. Different haplotypes share nucleotides and alleles at different locations and relative frequencies. LD between SNPs is misleading if used to define functional haplotypes. Haplospecific recombination creates further complexity [23,60,61].
7. There are at least two types of association with disease, as described above. No doubt, there will be further categories, especially as cis and trans interactions are defined. IDDM is an example of the need to address the mode of inheritance and multiple interactions, as described by Alper et al. [62,63]. Epistatic interactions may also be important.

8. The low positive predictive values of a genetic marker for a disease will remain so until the pathogenic pathways are understood. Fortunately, for clinical purposes, there are examples where the absence of an allele or sequence can be useful for the exclusion of a diagnosis. However, the presence of the same allele does not permit confirmation of the diagnosis—take, for example, HLA B27 [4]. Thus, those designing future studies should consider how the results will be of practical value, and at the same time, be useful in defining the biology.
9. Many regions of biological and statistical importance are not included in commercial SNP typing. In fact, duplications, indels, RLEs, and ambiguities may be very informative [16].
10. The MHC is a useful model for other genomic regions with polymorphic frozen blocks [64].
11. An understanding of synteny and paralogy is very valuable [65].
12. Many MHC associations, such as narcolepsy, 21-OH deficiency, and haemochromatosis are *not* immunologically mediated. There is no justification for prejudice in interpreting results. Current limited understanding of pathological processes may lead to confusion. In fact, as illustrated by the value of informative clinic-to-laboratory studies, there is potential to elucidate these processes.
13. A promising approach includes understanding the processes and genetics responsible for autoimmune diseases induced by immune checkpoint inhibitors, vaccines, and drugs, such as D-Penicillamine. The value of genomics increases when the inducing agent is known [15].

5. Conclusions

One lesson might be that there are incompatible concepts and terminology, as well as a very patchy understanding of the incontrovertible facts of MHC associations and structure. Another might be that research is constrained by the limitations of commercial platforms.

We hope our commentary is helpful in providing background for new discoveries. Hence the subtitle: "Looking Back to Go Forward". Surely, it is important not to dismiss the history as "HLA typing errors". In fact, the International HLA work-

shops provide a useful resource for haplotype association with disease, as well as for matching donors and hosts for transplantation.
SNP typing is most useful after the conserved ancestral haplotypes have been defined by other methods.

Funding: This research received no external funding.

Acknowledgments: We would like to thank Chester Alper, Jerzy Kulski, Michael Chorney, Ted Steele, Sue Lester, and the late Jon van Rood, for their encouragement and contributions to our understanding of this field. This is publication 1901 of the C Y O'Connor ERADE Village Foundation. Reference [5] is available on request.

Conflicts of interest: The authors declare no conflict of interest.

References

1. Brewerton, D.A.; Hart, F.D.; Nicholls, A.; Caffrey, M.; James, D.C.O.; Sturrock, R.D. Ankylosing Spondylitis and HL-A 27. *Lancet* **1973**, *301*, 904–907.
2. Schlosstein, L.; Terasaki, P.I.; Bluestone, R.; Pearson, C.M. High association of an HL-A antigen, W27, with ankylosing spondylitis. *N Engl J Med* **1973**, *288*, 704–706.
3. Dawkins, R.L.; Christiansen, F.T.; Zilko, P.J. Musculoskeletal Disease and D-penicillamine, including reports from the D-Pen - HLA 82 Workshop. *Immunogenet. Rheumatol.* **1982**.
4. Christiansen, F.T.; Hawkins, B.R.; Dawkins, R.L.; Owen, E.T.; Potter, R.M. The prevalence of ankylosing spondylitis among B27 positive normal individuals--a reassessment. *J. Rheumatol.* **1979**, *6*, 713–718.
5. Dawkins, R.L. *Adapting Genetics*; Near Urban Publishing: Dallas, TX, 2015; ISBN 978-0-9864115-1-9.
6. Brown, M.A.; Kenna, T.; Wordsworth, B.P. Genetics of ankylosing spondylitis - Insights into pathogenesis. *Nat. Rev. Rheumatol.* **2016**, *12*, 81–91.
7. Alper, C.A.; Awdeh, Z.L.; Raum, D.D.; Yunis, E.J. Extended major histocompatibility complex haplotypes in man: role of alleles analogous to murine t mutants. *Clin Immunol Immunopathol* **1982**, *24*, 276–285.
8. Dawkins, R.L.; Christiansen, F.T.; Kay, P.H.; Garlepp, M.; McCluskey, J.; Hollingsworth, P.N.; Zilko, P.J. Disease associations with complotypes, supratypes and haplotypes. *Immunol. Rev.* **1983**, *70*, 5–22.
9. Rigby, R.J.; Dawkins, R.L.; Wetherall, J.D.; Hawkins, B.R. HLA in systemic lupus erythematosus: influence on severity. *Tissue Antigens* **1978**, *12*, 25–31.

10. Christiansen, F.T.; Dawkins, R.L.; Uko, G.; McCluskey, J.; Kay, P.H.; Zilko, P.J. Complement allotyping in SLE: association with C4A null. *Aust. N. Z. J. Med.* **1983**, *13*, 483–488.
11. Chabas, D.; Taheri, S.; Renier, C.; Mignot, E. The Genetics of Narcolepsy. *Annu. Rev. Genomics Hum. Genet.* **2003**, *4*, 459–483.
12. Hollingsworth, P.N.; Dawkins, R.L.; Peter, J.B. HLA and narcolepsy. *Neurology* **1993**, *43*, 1444–1445.
13. Gerhard, G.S.; Ten Elshof, A.E.; Chorney, M.J. Hereditary haemochromatosis as an immunological disease. *Br. J. Haematol.* **1998**, *100*, 247–255.
14. Feder, J.N.; Gnirke, A.; Thomas, W.; Tsuchihashi, Z.; Ruddy, D.A.; Basava, A.; Dormishian, F.; Domingo Jr., R.; Ellis, M.C.; Fullan, A.; et al. A novel MHC class I-like gene is mutated in patients with hereditary haemochromatosis. *Nat. Genet.* **1996**, *13*, 399–408.
15. Mallal, S.; Nolan, D.; Witt, C.; Masel, G.; Martin, A.M.; Moore, C.; Sayer, D.; Castley, A.; Mamotte, C.; Maxwell, D.; et al. Association between presence of HLA-B*5701, HLA-DR7, and HLA-DQ3 and hypersensitivity to HIV-1 reverse-transcriptase inhibitor abacavir. *Lancet* **2002**, *359*, 727–732.
16. Dawkins, R.L.; Leelayuwat, C.; Gaudieri, S.; Tay, G.; Hui, J.; Cattley, S.; Martinez, P.; Kulski, J. Genomics of the major histocompatibility complex: haplotypes, duplication, retroviruses and disease. *Immunol. Rev.* **1999**, *167*, 275–304.
17. McCluskey, J.; Kay, P.H.; Stickey, M.; Christiansen, F.T.; Dawkins, R.L.; Wilson, G. MHC "supratype" predicting heterozygous 21-hydroxylase deficiency. *Lancet* **1983**, *1*, 764–765.
18. White, P.C.; New, M.I.; Dupont, B. HLA-linked congenital adrenal hyperplasia results from a defective gene encoding a cytochrome P-450 specific for steroid 21-hydroxylation. *Proc. Natl. Acad. Sci.* **1984**, *81*, 7505–7509.
19. Raum, D.; Awdeh, Z.; Yunis, E.J.; Alper, C.A.; Gabbay, K.H. Extended major histocompatibility complex haplotypes in type I diabetes mellitus. *J. Clin. Invest.* **1984**, *74*, 449–454.
20. Alper, C.A.; Larsen, C.E. Major Histocompatibility Complex: Disease Associations. In *eLS*; John Wiley & Sons, Ltd.: Chichester., 2015; pp. 1–8 ISBN 9780470015902.
21. Gaudieri, S.; Leelayuwat, C.; Tay, G.K.; Townend, D.C.; Dawkins, R.L. The major histocompatibility complex (MHC) contains conserved polymorphic genomic sequences that are shuffled by recombination to form ethnic-specific haplotypes. *J. Mol. Evol.* **1997**, *45*, 17–23.
22. Lam, T.H.; Tay, M.Z.; Wang, B.; Xiao, Z.; Ren, E.C. Intrahaplotypic variants differentiate complex linkage disequilibrium within human MHC haplotypes. *Sci. Rep.* **2015**, *5*, 1–16.
23. Carrington, M. Recombination within the human MHC. *Immunol. Rev.* **1999**, *167*, 245–256.
24. Christiansen, F.T.; Pollack, M.S.; Garlepp, M.J.; Dawkins, R.L. Myasthenia gravis and HLA antigens in American blacks and other races. *J. Neuroimmunol.* **1984**, *7*, 121–129.

25. Todd, J.A.; Mijovic, C.; Fletcher, J.; Jenkins, D.; Bradwell, A.R.; Barnett, A.H. Identification of susceptibility loci for insulin-dependent diabetes mellitus by trans-racial gene mapping. *Nature* **1989**, *338*, 587–589.
26. Alper, C.A.; Larsen, C.E.; Dubey, D.P.; Awdeh, Z.L.; Fici, D.A.; Yunis, E.J. The Haplotype Structure of the Human Major Histocompatibility Complex. *Hum. Immunol.* **2006**, *67*, 73–84.
27. Degli-Esposti, M.A.; Andreas, A.; Christiansen, F.T.; Schalke, B.; Albert, E.; Dawkins, R.L. An approach to the localization of the susceptibility genes for generalized myasthenia gravis by mapping recombinant ancestral haplotypes. *Immunogenetics* **1992**, *35*, 355–364.
28. Kelly, H.; McCann, V.J.; Kay, P.H.; Dawkins, R.L. Susceptibility to IDDM is marked by MHC supratypes rather than individual alleles. *Immunogenetics* **1985**, *22*, 643–651.
29. Fernando, M.M.; Stevens, C.R.; Sabeti, P.C.; Walsh, E.C.; McWhinnie, A.J.; Shah, A.; Green, T.; Rioux, J.D.; Vyse, T.J. Identification of two independent risk factors for lupus within the MHC in United Kingdom families. *PLoS Genet* **2007**, *3*, e192.
30. Pugliese, A.; Gianani, R.; Moromisato, R.; Awdeh, Z.L.; Alper, C.A.; Erlich, H.A.; Jackson, R.A.; Eisenbarth, G.S. HLA-DQB1*0602 is associated with dominant protection from diabetes even among islet cell antibody-positive first-degree relatives of patients with IDDM. *Diabetes* **1995**, *44*, 608–613.
31. Schloot, N.C.; Roep, B.O.; Wegmann, D.; Yu, L.; Chase, H.P.; Wang, T.; Eisenbarth, G.S. Altered immune response to insulin in newly diagnosed compared to insulin-treated diabetic patients and healthy control subjects. *Diabetologia* **1997**, *40*, 564–572.
32. Rewers, M.; Norris, J.M.; Eisenbarth, G.S.; Erlich, H.A.; Beaty, B.; Klingensmith, G.; Hoffman, M.; Yu, L.; Bugawan, T.L.; Blair, A.; et al. Beta-cell autoantibodies in infants and toddlers without IDDM relatives: Diabetes autoimmunity study in the young (DAISY). *J. Autoimmun.* **1996**, *9*, 405–410.
33. Dawkins, R.L.; Willamson, J.F.; Lester, S.; Dawkins, S.T. Mutation versus polymorphism in evolution. *Genomics* **2013**, *101*, 211–212.
34. Dawkins, R.L.; Leaver, A.; Cameron, P.U.; Martin, E.; Kay, P.H.; Christiansen, F.T. Some disease-associated ancestral haplotypes carry a polymorphism of TNF. *Hum. Immunol.* **1989**, *26*, 91–97.
35. Degli-Esposti, M.A.; Leaver, A.L.; Frank, T.; Witt, C.S.; Abraham, L.J.; Dawkins, R.L. Ancestral Haplotypes: Conserved Population MHC Haplotypes. *Hum. Immunol.* **1992**, *34*, 242–252.
36. Kennedy, A.E.; Ozbek, U.; Dorak, M.T. What has GWAS done for HLA and disease associations? International Journal of Immunogenetics, 44(5), 195–211. https://doi.org/10.1111/iji.12332 has GWAS done for HLA and disease associations? *Int. J. Immunogenet.* **2017**, *44*, 195–211.
37. Ceppellini, R.; Curtoni, E.S.; Mattuiz, P.L.; V.Miggiano; Scudeller, G.; Serra, A. Genetics of Leukocyte Antigens: A Family Study of Segregation and Linkage. In *Histocompatibility Testing 1967*; Curtoni, E.S., Mattiuz,

P.L., Tosi, R.M., Eds.; Munksgaard, Copenhagen, 1967; pp. 149–187.
38. Petersdorf, E.W. In celebration of Ruggero Ceppellini: HLA in transplantation. *HLA* **2017**, *89*, 71–76.
39. Manolio, T.A.; Brooks, L.D.; Collins, F.S. A HapMap harvest of insights into the genetics of common disease. *Fournal Clin. Investig.* **2008**, *118*, 1590–1605.
40. International HapMap Consortium A haplotype map of the human genome. *Nature* **2005**, *437*, 1299–320.
41. International HapMap Consortium The International HapMap Project. *Nature* **2003**, *426*, 789–796.
42. Ka, S.; Lee, S.; Hong, J.; Cho, Y.; Sung, J.; Kim, H.N.; Kim, H.L.; Jung, J. HLAscan: Genotyping of the HLA region using next-generation sequencing data. *BMC Bioinformatics* **2017**, *18*, 1–12.
43. Gaudieri, S.; Dawkins, R.L.; Habara, K.; Kulski, J.K.; Gojobori, T. SNP profile within the Human Major Histocompatibility Complex reveals an extreme and interrupted level of nucleotide diversity. *Genome Res.* **2000**, *10*, 1579–1586.
44. Longman-Jacobsen, N.; Williamson, J.F.; Dawkins, R.L.; Gaudieri, S. In Polymorphic Genomic Regions Indels Cluster with Nucleotide Polymorphism: Quantum Genomics. *Gene* **2003**, *312*, 257–261.
45. Romero, V.; Larsen, C.E.; Duke-Cohan, J.S.; Fox, E.A.; Romero, T.; Clavijo, O.P.; Fici, D.A.; Husain, Z.; Almeciga, I.; Alford, D.R.; et al. Genetic fixity in the human major histocompatibility complex and block size diversity in the class I region including HLA-E. *BMC Genet* **2007**, *8*, 14.
46. Gabriel, S.B.; Schaffner, S.F.; Nguyen, H.; Moore, J.M.; Blumenstiel, B.; Higgins, J.; Defelice, M.; Lochner, A.; Faggart, M.; Liu-cordero, S.N.; et al. The Structure of Haplotype Blocks in the Human Genome. *Science* **2002**, *296*, 2225–2229.
47. Petersdorf, E.W.; O'hUigin, C. The MHC in the era of next-generation sequencing: Implications for bridging structure with function. *Hum. Immunol.* **2019**, *80*, 67–78.
48. Abraham, L.J.; French, M.A.; Dawkins, R.L. Polymorphic MHC ancestral haplotypes affect the activity of tumour necrosis factor-alpha. *Clin. Exp. Immunol.* **1993**, *92*, 14–18.
49. Wilton, A.N.; Cobain, T.J.; Dawkins, R.L. Family studies of IgA deficiency. *Immunogenetics* **1985**, *21*, 333–342.
50. Tay, G.K.; Witt, C.S.; Christiansen, F.T.; Charron, D.; Baker, D.; Herrmann, R.; Smith, L.K.; Diepeveen, D.; Mallal, S.; McCluskey, J.; et al. Matching for MHC haplotypes results in improved survival following unrelated bone marrow transplantation. *Bone Marrow Transplant.* **1995**, *15*, 381–385.
51. Wilton, A.N.; Christiansen, F.T.; Dawkins, R.L. Supratype matching improves renal transplantation survival. *Transplant. Proc.* **1985**, *17*, 2211–2216.
52. Vadva, Z.; Larsen, C.E.; Propp, B.E.; Trautwein, M.R.; Alford, D.R.; Alper, C.A. A New Pedigree-Based SNP Haplotype Method for Genomic Poly-

morphism and Genetic Studies. *Cells* **2019**, *8*, 1–17.

53. Lloyd, S.S.; Steele, E.J.; Dawkins, R.L. Analysis of Haplotype Sequences. In *Next Generation Sequencing - Advances, Applications and Challenges*; Kulski, J.K., Ed.; InTech, 2016; pp. 345–368 ISBN 978-953-51-2240-1.
54. Horton, R.; Gibson, R.; Coggill, P.; Miretti, M.; Allcock, R.J.; Almeida, J.; Forbes, S.; Gilbert, J.G.R.; Halls, K.; Harrow, J.L.; et al. Variation analysis and gene annotation of eight MHC haplotypes: the MHC Haplotype Project. *Immunogenetics* **2008**, *60*, 1–18.
55. Jensen, J.M.; Villesen, P.; Friborg, R.M.; Mailund, T.; Besenbacher, S.; Schierup, M.H. Assembly and analysis of 100 full MHC haplotypes from the Danish population. *Genome Res.* **2017**, *27*, 1597–1607.
56. Alper, C.A.; Larsen, C.E. Pedigree-Defined Haplotypes and Their Applications to Genetic Studies. In *Haplotyping: Methods and Protocols, Methods in Molecular Biology*; 2008; Vol. 1551, pp. 113–127 ISBN 9781493967506.
57. International Histocompatibility Working Group, Available online: http://www.ihwg.org/ (accessed on: 19 August 2019).
58. Norman, P.J.; Norberg, S.J.; Guethlein, L.A.; Nemat-Gorgani, N.; Royce, T.; Wroblewski, E.E.; Dunn, T.; Mann, T.; Alicata, C.; Hollenbach, J.A.; et al. Sequences of 95 human MHC haplotypes reveal extreme coding variation in genes other than highly polymorphic HLA class i and II. *Genome Res.* **2017**, *27*, 813–823.
59. Kasahara, M. The chromosomal duplication model of the major histocompatibility complex. *Immunol. Rev.* **1999**, *167*, 17–32.
60. van Oosterhout, C. Trans-species polymorphism, HLA-disease associations and the evolution of the MHC. *Commun Integr Biol* **2009**, *2*, 408–410.
61. Ahmad, T.; Neville, M.; Marshall, S.E.; Armuzzi, A.; Mulcahy-Hawes, K.; Crawshaw, J.; Sato, H.; Ling, K.L.; Barnardo, M.; Goldthorpe, S.; et al. Haplotype-specific linkage disequilibrium patterns define the genetic topography of the human MHC. *Hum. Mol. Genet.* **2003**, *12*, 647–656.
62. Aly, T.A.; Eller, E.; Ide, A.; Gowan, K.; Babu, S.R.; Erlich, H.A.; Rewers, M.J.; Eisenbarth, G.S.; Fain, P.R. Multi-SNP analysis of MHC region: remarkable conservation of HLA-A1-B8-DR3 haplotype. *Diabetes* **2006**, *55*, 1265–1269.
63. Hutton, J.C.; Eisenbarth, G.S. A pancreatic β-cell-specific homolog of glucose-6-phosphatase emerges as a major target of cell-mediated autoimmunity in diabetes. *Proc. Natl. Acad. Sci.* **2003**, *100*, 8626–8628.
64. McLure, C.A.; Hinchliffe, P.; Lester, S.; Williamson, J.F.; Millman, J.A.; Keating, P.J.; Stewart, B.J.; Dawkins, R.L. Genomic evolution and polymorphism: Segmental duplications and haplotypes at 108 regions on 21 chromosomes. *Genomics* **2013**, *102*, 15–26.
65. Dawkins, R.L.; Berry, J.; Martinez, P.; Gaudieri, S.; Hui, J.; Cattley, S.; Longman, N.; Kulski, J.; Carnegie, P. Potential for Paralogous Mapping to Simplify the Genetics of Diseases and Functions Associated with MHC Haplotypes. In *The Major Histocompatibility Complex: Evolution, Structure, and Function*; Kasahara, M., Ed.; Springer-Verlag Tokyo, 2000; pp146–157.

Interspecies Translation: Bovine Marbling to Human Muscular Dystrophy

Jose L. Valenzuela, Sally S. Lloyd, Edward J. Steele, Francis L. Mastaglia and Roger L. Dawkins
Published by InTech, in the book Muscular Dystrophy, editor Kunihiro Sakuma
DOI: http://dx.doi.org/10.5772/intechopen.82685

Abstract
There are interesting similarities and differences when comparing the histopathology of bovine marbling and human muscular dystrophy. At the simplest level, both conditions are characterized by genetically controlled and more or less inexorable replacement of muscle fibers with fat cells. At issue is whether an improved understanding of these two processes can lead to better outcomes for patients. There are many forms of dystrophy that differ in their genetics and their histopathology. There are also many forms of "marbling" ranging from the coarse to fine, epimysial, perimysial to endomysial and even to total replacement or steatosis. A detailed examination of marbling will provide a framework for further investigation of human dystrophy. Ultimately, the many genetic factors involved can be addressed through a better understanding of the metabolic pathways involved in marbling.
Keywords: synteny, muscular dystrophy, bovine marbling, adipogenesis

1. Introduction
The purpose of this review is to compare the genetics and histopathology of bovine marbling and human muscular dystrophy. Surprisingly, in spite of similarities, the literature suggests that marbling is a function of extreme adipogenesis whereas dystrophy is a consequence of fundamental defects in muscle itself. In fact, completely independent studies, as summarized here, reveal that similar genes have been implicated in some selected situations. Further, it is clear that the histopathology of some forms of dystrophy can resemble some forms of bovine marbling.

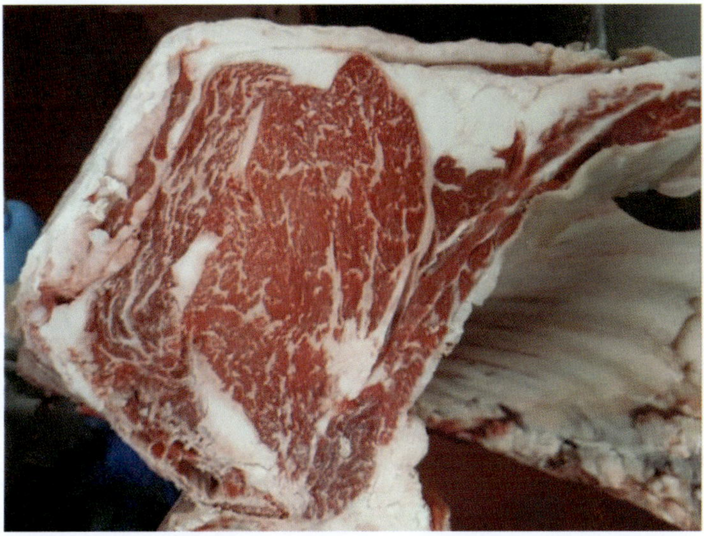

Figure 1. Loin at the 11th intercostal level of carcase of Melaleuka Stud steer M508 (wy63 ak25 dx13), MSA MB 1100, DOF 471. There are extensive areas of fine marbling as indicated by pink muscle with fine flecks. Note 88% wagyu (63% black, 25% red Akaushi). See also Figure 5 for microscopic features.

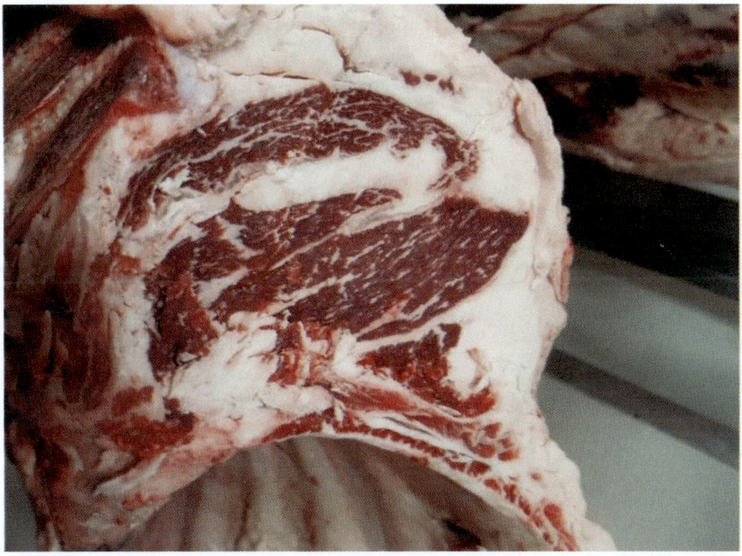

Figure 2. Loin at the 11th intercostal level of carcase of Melaleuka Stud heifer M621 (wy75 dx25), MSA MB 920, DOF 443. There is a predominance of fat arborizing from the subcutaneous tissue and creating coarse marbling. The muscle areas are dark red in comparison to Fig.1. Note lower MSA MB of 920 but similar days on feed (DOF).

2. Marbling

Marbling is the term used to describe the presence of macroscopically visible fat within muscle (**Figures 1** and **2**). Coarse marbling refers to white areas of fat through and around muscle bundles, generally as continuous bands arising from the subcutaneous adipose tissue. By contrast, fine or "snowflake" marbling is characterized
by more even white flecks resulting in pink rather than red muscle.

These two forms may coexist but can be distinguished and quantified by skilled observers. Fine marbling is associated with improved taste and tenderness [1]. Further, it has been shown to relate to a preferred fatty acid profile. Accordingly, there is copious funding and now a substantial understanding of the environmental and genetic factors which favor fine rather than coarse.

3. Interspecies translation

Interspecies translation from cattle to man has unrecognized potential. Firstly, cattle are close to humans in evolutionary time and fall within that window of 50–100 million years of separation (or last common ancestor) which is characterized by very similar proteins but vastly different regulations of expression. The same window may explain the fact that the two species have synergized over some 40,000 years of contact and at least 7000 years of domestication. As one example, infections can be similar and, in some cases, are transmissible from one to the other, but close exposure to cattle is generally innocuous implying some form of immunity. As for example in the case of pox and tuberculosis. We argue that cattle are both relevant and relatively safe for translational studies.

Secondly, domestic cattle are well maintained, closely observed, and very well understood. There are huge databases and DNA banks which have been in existence for 50 years. Innumerable breeds can be compared often under different environmental conditions. Many of these breeds have been closed for hundreds of years and then intentionally crossed with each other. There is great potential for meaningful studies of population genetics and family and haplotype associations and, even more so, for structure-function genomics. Metabolic and inflammatory

pathways are relatively well understood and are supported by inestimable funding available to ensure future supplies of meat, milk, cheese, butter, leather, and fertilizer.
Thirdly, cattle are plentiful and even more so than humans. Because the generation time and life expectancy are much shorter, there are excellent opportunities to study and treat genetically determined diseases prospectively [2].

4. Other instances of translation

White muscle disease or selenium/vitamin E deficiency occurs quite commonly in livestock raised on leached soils. The pathology resembles dystrophy in some respects. A mutation in the selenoprotein N gene (SEPN1) is responsible for some types of congenital muscular dystrophies and myopathies [3]. Kakulas [4] demonstrated that dystrophy-like changes explained the weakness observed in quokkas on Rottnest Island. Importantly, the condition could be corrected by treating the deficiency raising the possibility that human dystrophies could be reversible if the basic defect could be corrected.

5. Genomic approach

The term genome is used here to refer to the architecture of DNA sequences, whereas others have come to use the term in the context of single-nucleotide polymorphisms wherever they occur. The difference is fundamental to the discovery of gene clusters with coherent cis and trans interactions between conserved sequences known as ancestral haplotypes [5–9]. Many studies have shown that the SNP approach in livestock and humans fails to identify these critical sequences and can be misleading at best [10]. SNPs are neutral markers of parentage rather than functionally important [11]. One major benefit of ancestral haplotypes as opposed to SNPs is that it is possible to use interspecies translation. During mammalian evolution, polymorphic frozen blocks have diverged to some extent although the functionally important sequences tend to be conserved. As shown in **Figure 3** and **Table 1**, there are similarities between genomic regions on Hosa 17 and Bota 19. Although there have been architectural changes such as insertions and transversions, the gene content has been preserved. Bota 19 was chosen as the reference because of its critical role in determining the degree of marbling between individuals of a breed, F1 crosses and between breeds [5, 12–14].

Hosa 17 was chosen for comparison because it contains some of the same genes such as TCAP. Further analysis revealed an extraordinary degree of preservation or synteny in spite of an evolutionary separation time of at least 50 million years and therefore millions of generations. Implicit is that there are functional reasons for similarities in genomic architecture.
Yet further analysis suggests some explanations for the co-location of similar genes. Irrespective of cis and trans interactions between the protein products, there is evidence of co-regulation (see, e.g., SREBP). In this context, we conclude that, although products and their regulating transcription factors are preserved, separation has permitted the insertion of species-specific elements, which control the quantitative differences between humans and cattle.
Importantly, as shown in **Figure 3** and **Table 1**, Hosa 17 contains multiple candidates for involvement in human muscular dystrophy. There is even more complexity in explaining the multiple candidates as shown in **Tables 2** and **3**. Thus, syntenic analysis has suggested a novel approach to identification of operative elements in marbling and in some forms of

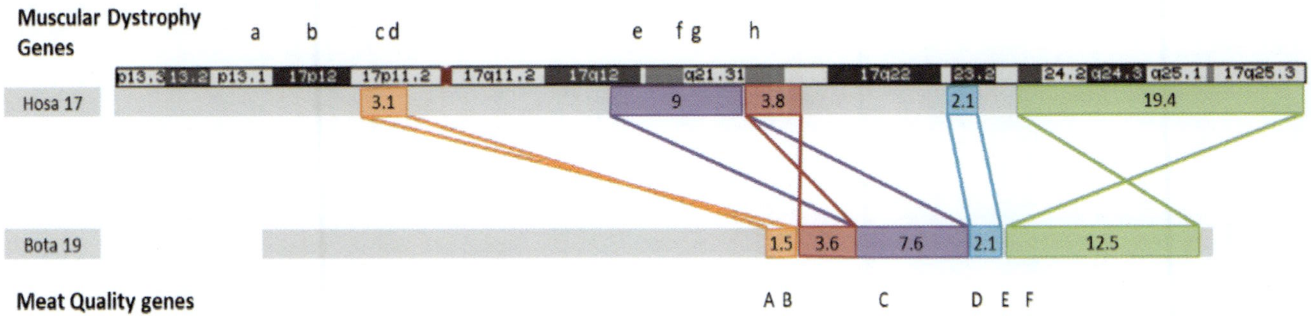

Figure 3. Marbling and muscular dystrophy are syntenic on bovine chromosome 19 (Bota 19) and human chromosome 17 (Hosa 17). Colored boxes represent segments with the same gene content. Crossed joining lines indicate inverted translocations. Numbers represent Mb. Synteny was determined by the positions of homologous genes in the human assembly Hg 38 and bovine assembly BosTau8 located using the UCSC genome browser. Inverted sections and the exact location of boundaries between blocks were determined by dotplots comparing the two sequences. Adapted from: [13] Locations of **Muscular Dystrophy Genes**: (a) MYH2, (b) PMP22, (c) TRPV2, (d) SREBF1, (e) TCAP, (f) CAVIN1, (g) BECN1, (h) SGCA and **Meat Quality Genes** (A)SREBF1, (B) MPRIP, (C) TCAP, (D) GH, (E) UTS2R, (F) FASN shown here. See **Table 1** for more information about these genes.

Table 1.
Details of relevant genes in Bota 19 and Hosa 17.

GENE Location	**Description**	**Human muscular Dystrophy**	**Meat Quality Trait**
MYH2 Hosa 17p13.1 Bota chr19: 30.13Mb	MYH2 encodes the myosin heavy chain isoform that is expressed in fast type 2A muscle fibers	proximal myopathy and ophthalmoplegia	In pork, IMF, water holding capacity, and meat color.[18]
PMP22 Hosa 17p12 Bota chr19: 33.35Mb	peripheral myelin protein-22	Duplication of this gene causes Charcot-Marie-Tooth disease type 1A	
TRPV2 Hosa 17p11.2 Bota chr19: 33.816Mb	Transient Receptor Potential cation Channel, V2: Responds to heat and cations	Muscular dystrophy is ameliorated in dystrophin-deficient mdx mice by dominant-negative inhibition of TRPV2 [19]	
SREBF1 Hosa 17p11.2 Bota chr19: 35.23Mb	Sterol regulatory element-binding protein-1 controls cholesterol homeostasis by stimulating transcription of sterol-regulated genes	Mutations of LMNA that cause Emery-Dreifuss muscular dystrophy (EDMD2-AD) and familial partial lipodystrophy (FPLD2) result in less binding of lamin A to SREBP1. [20]	Alleles of SREBF1 are associated with fatty acid composition of Japanese Black Cattle[21]
MPRIP Hosa 17p11.2 Bota chr19: 35.56Mb	Myosin phosphatase rho-interacting protein. regulates the phosphorylation of myosin light chain		

Table 1. continued
Details of relevant genes in Bota 19 and Hosa 17.

GENE Location	Description	Human muscular Dystrophy	Meat Quality Trait
SGCA Hosa 17q21.33 Bota chr19: 37.11Mb	Sarcoglycan, alpha Sarcoglycans form part of the dystrophin-glycoprotein complex.	Mutations in SGCA cause Limb-girdle muscular dystrophy type 2D. SGCB, SGCD and SGCG are associated with LGMD types 2E, 2F and 2C respectively. [22]	
TCAP Hosa 17q12 Bota chr19: 40.69Mb	Titin-Cap (telethonin) is a sarcomeric protein localized to the periphery of Z discs that define the border of the sarcomere as a structural anchor and signaling center.	Limb-girdle muscular dystrophy type 2G (LGMD2G) is caused by mutations in the TCAP gene[23]	TCAP indel associated with marble score in Hanwoo Cattle [24]
CAVIN1 Hosa 17q21.2 Bota chr19: 43.14 Mb	CAVIN is an essential factor in the biogenesis of caveolae	Congenital generalized lipodystrophy, type 4; (CGL4) is caused by mutations in CAVIN1 that result in CAV 3 deficiency.	
BECN1 Hosa 17q21.31 Bota chr19: 43.47Mb	Beclin-1 participates in the regulation of autophagy	Expression of BECN1 was reduced in patients with muscular dystrophies BTHLM1 and UMCD1 which were caused by COL6A1 mutations.	Involved in Proteolysis, beef aging.[25]

Table 1. continued
Details of relevant genes in Bota 19 and Hosa 17.

GENE Location	Description	Human muscular Dystrophy	Meat Quality Trait
GH1 Hosa 17q23.3 Bota Chr19: 48.77Mb	Growth Hormone		A polymorphism of growth hormone is associated with fatty acid composition of Wagyu beef [32]
FASN Hosa 17q25.3 Bota Chr19: 51.38 Mb	Fatty Acid Synthase the key enzyme of de novo lipogenesis to produce saturated fatty acids		Fatty Acid Synthase is highlighted in GWAS for fatty acid content and composition of Wagyu and Hanwoo beef [33, 34]
UTS2R Hosa17q25.3 Bota Chr19: 50.81 Mb	A receptor abundant in heart and pancreas and responsive to Urotensin II which has potent vasoactive properties		A polymorphism of UTS2R is associated with IMF content of Wagyu x Holstein beef [39]

Table 2.

Details of relevant genes outside of Hosa 17/Bota 19.

Gene location	Description	Human muscular dystrophy	Meat quality trait
MSTN Hosa 2q32.2 Bota chr2: 6.21Mb	Myostatin	Muscle hypertrophy was caused by a homozygous mutation in myostatin [35]	Mutations in myostatin cause double muscling in several cattle breeds [36]
CAPN3 Hosa 15q15.1 Bota chr10: 37.8Mb	Calpains are nonlysosomal intracellular cysteine proteases. CAPN3 is a muscle-specific large subunit	Limb-girdle muscular dystrophy type 2A (LGMD2A) is caused by homozygous or compound heterozygous mutation in CAPN3	SNPs within CAPN3 are associated with tenderness in *Bos Indicus* cattle [37]
CAPN1 Hosa 11q13.1 Bota chr29: 44.06Mb	m-Calpain		Two CAPN1 genetic markers are associated with tenderness in Brahman beef [38]
DMD Hosa Xp21.2-.1 Bota chrX: 115.34Mb	Dystrophin maintains the structural integrity of myofibrils	Duchene muscular dystrophy	
LAMA2 Hosa 6q22.33 Bota chr9: 67.96Mb	LAMA2 gene encodes the alpha-2 chain of laminin-2 Laminin-2 (merosin) is the main laminin found in muscle fibers	Congenital merosin-deficient muscular dystrophy type 1A; MDC1A	

Table 2. continued

Details of relevant genes outside of Hosa 17/Bota 19.

Gene location	Description	Human muscular dystrophy	Meat quality trait
MYOT Hosa 5q31.2 Bota chr7: 50.94Mb	Myotilin directly binds F-actin and efficiently cross-links actin filaments and prevents filament disassembly	LGMD1A is caused by heterozygous mutation in the MYOT. It is characterized by adult-onset muscle weakness, progressing from the hip to the shoulder girdle	SNPs in MYOT correlate with loin muscle area and intramuscular fat in Qinchuan cattle[39]
CAV3 Hosa 3p25.3 Bota chr22: 17.83Mb	Caveolin 3	Muscular dystrophy, limb-girdle, type 1C; LGMD1C	
SGCD Hosa 5q33.2-.3 Bota chr7: 69.59Mb	Sarcoglycan, delta is expressed in skeletal and heart muscles and to a lesser extent in smooth muscle. Delta-sarcoglycan is localized at the sarcolemma	Muscular dystrophy, limb-girdle, type 2F; LGMD2F	
SGCE Hosa 7q21.3 Bota chr4: 11.84Mb	Epsilon-sarcoglycan	Myoclonus-dystonia is a genetically heterogeneous disorder characterized by myoclonic jerks affecting mostly proximal muscles	

Table 2. continued

Details of relevant genes outside of Hosa 17/Bota 19.

Gene location	Description	Human muscular dystrophy	Meat quality trait
SGCB Bota chr6: 69.53Mb	Beta-sarcoglycan		
SGCG at Bota chr12: 34.92Mb			
COL6A1 COL6A2 21q22.3	Collagen, type VI, alpha-1, and alpha-2 Members of the collagen VI family form distinct net-works of microfibrils in connective tissue and interact with other extracellular matrix components	Ullrich congenital muscular dystrophy 1 Bethlem myopathy 1	
COL6A3 2q37.3	COLLAGEN, TYPE VI, ALPHA-3	Ullrich congenital muscular dystrophy 1, Bethlem myopathy 1 Dystonia 27	
ITGA7 12q13.2	The alpha-7 integrin is a specific cellular receptor for the basement membrane proteins laminin-1, laminin-2, and laminin-4. The alpha-7 subunit is expressed mainly in skeletal and cardiac muscles and may be involved in differentiation and migration processes during myogenesis	Congenital muscular dystrophy	
EMD Xq28	Emerin is found along the nuclear rim of many cell types and is a member of the nuclear lamina-associated protein family	Emery-dreifuss muscular dystrophy 1, X-LINKED; EDMD1	

Table 2. continued

Details of relevant genes outside of Hosa 17/Bota 19.

Gene location	Description	Human muscular dystrophy	Meat quality trait
ATP2A1 (SERCA-1) 16p11.2	Calcium-transporting ATPase lower cytoplasmic Ca(2+) concentration by pumping Ca(2+) to luminal or extracellular spaces. ATP2A1 is the ATPase type found in fast twitch muscles	Brody myopathy	
DES 2q35	Desmin is the muscle-specific member of the intermediate filament (IF) protein family. It is one of the earliest myogenic markers, both in the heart and somites, and is expressed in satellite stem cells and replicating myoblasts	Myopathy, myofibrillar, 1	
PLEC 8q24.3	Plectin-1 is one of the largest polypeptides known and is believed to provide mechanical strength to cells and tissues by acting as a cross-linking element of the cytoskeleton	Epidermolysis bullosa with muscular dystrophy Limb-girdle type 2Q	

Table 3. Protein accumulations and deficits in dystrophy.

(Adapted from [15] Table 6.3).

Absent protein	Dystrophy type	Gene location
Dystrophin	Xp21 muscular dystrophies (Duchenne, Becker)	DMD Hosa Xp21.2-p21.1 Bota X
Sarcoglycans	Limb-girdle muscular dystrophies 2C-F	SGCA Bota 19 Hosa 17q21.33 SGCB Bota 6 SGCD Bota 7 Hosa 5q33.2 SGCE Bota 4 Hosa 7q21.3 SGCG Bota 12
Dysferlin	Limb-girdle muscular dystrophy 2B	DYSF Hosa 2p13.2
Caveolin-3	Limb-girdle muscular dystrophy 1a, rippling muscle disease, hyperCKemia	CAV3 Hosa 3p25.3 Bota 22 CAVIN1 Hosa 17q21.2 Bota 19
Telethonin	Limb-girdle muscular dystrophy 2G	TCAP Hosa 17q12 Bota 19
Laminin a2	MDC1A ("merosin"-deficient congenital muscular dystrophy)	LAMA2 Hosa 6q22.33, Bota 9
Collagen VI	Ullrich congenital muscular dystrophy	COL6A1&2 Hosa 21q22.3 COL6A3 Hosa 2q37.3
Integrin alpha7	Mild congenital dystrophy/myopathy	ITGA7 Hosa 12q13.2
Calpain-3 (easier to assess on immunoblots than sections)	Limb-girdle muscular dystrophy 2A	CAPN3 Hosa 15q15.1 Bota 10
Emerin	X-Linked emery-dreifuss muscular dystrophy	EMD Hosa Xq28
SERCA 1	Brody disease	**ATP2A1 Hosa 16p11.2**
Plectin	Epidermolysis bullosa with muscular dystrophy, limb-girdle dystrophy 2Q	PLEC Hosa 8q24.3
LAMP-2	Danon disease	LAMP2 Xq24
Accumulating protein	Dystrophy type	Gene location
Actin	Congenital actin myopathy/nemaline myopathy	ACTA1 Hosa 1q24.13 TPM3 Hosa 1q23
Myosin	Myosin storage myopathy	MYH7 Hosa 14q11
Myotilin	Myotilin-related myofibrillar myopathy	MYOT Hosa 5q31.2
Desmin	Desmin myopathy	DES Hosa 2q35 SEPN1 Hosa

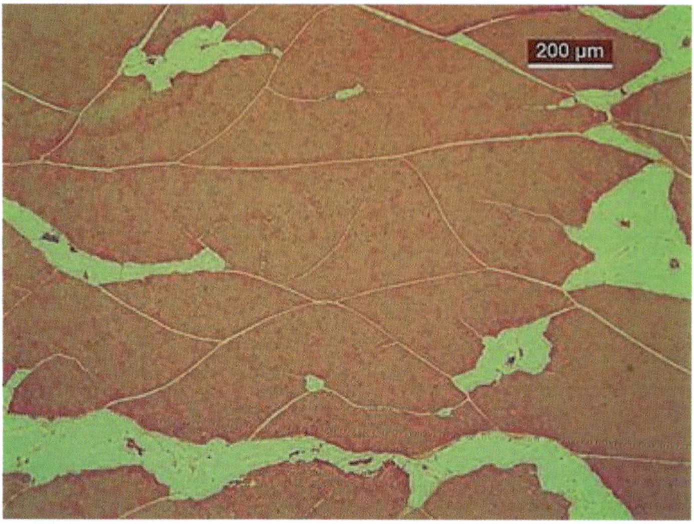

Figure 4. Highly marbled loin muscle shows a pattern of fat arborization and invasion with adipocytes predominantly in the perimysium, between muscle fascicles. Note extensive vascularization centrally within the fat. M508 (wy63 ak25 dx13), MSA MB 1100, DOF 471. See also Figure 1.

1p36

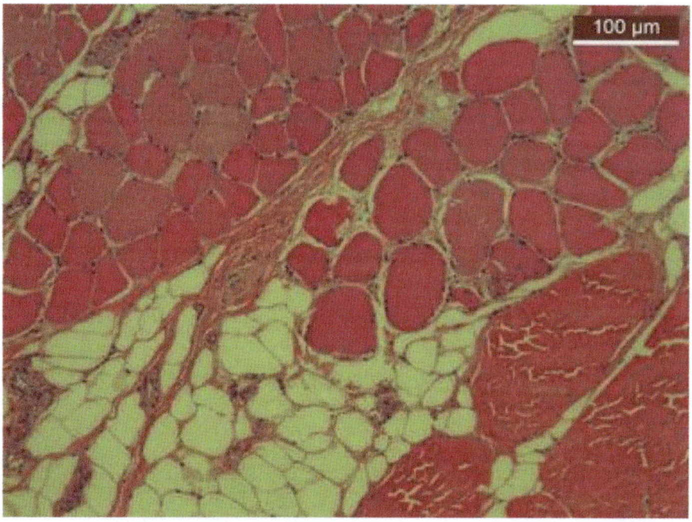

Figure 5. Histological section of Sacrocaudalis dorsalis medialis of a highly marbled, high Wagyu content (88%) steer M508 (wy63 ak25 dx13), showing variation of fiber size, with the presence of rounded fibers, internal nuclei, abundant perimysial connective tissue, and considerable adipose tissue. Formalin-fixed H & E, MSA MB 1100, DOF 471. CYO lab number Ch18/110G. See also Figure 1 for macroscopic comparison.

6. Histopathological approach

The substantial range of changes found in the human dystrophies is illustrated in the study of Dubowitz et al. [15].

We are fortunate in having histological muscle samples from cattle with degrees of marbling [14]. Some of these changes are illustrated in Figures 4, 5, 6, 7, 8 from three animals (M508, M621, and M129) fed a standard ration for 471, 443, and 481 days respectively.

The macroscopic measure of marbling (MSA MB) ranged from high to moderate (1100, 920 and 820, respectively) as expected in high content Wagyu (88, 75, and 63%, respectively). A common feature is the invasion of adipose tissue between intact muscle fascicles (Figure 4). For the most part, the process extends along the perimysium leading to variation in fiber size, staining of myofibers (Figures 5 and 6), and the formation of residual islands of myofibers (Figure 7), which suggests an explanation for fine (see Figure 1) rather than coarse (see Figure 2) marbling; fine is due to more aggressive invasion reflecting quantitative differences in gene regulation.

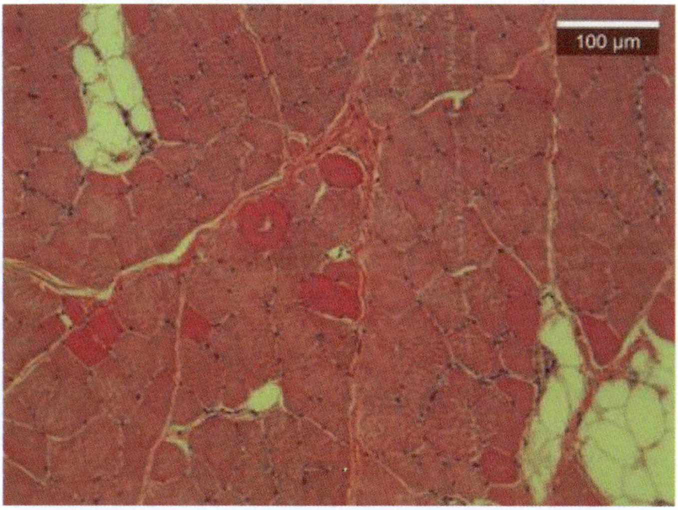

Figure 6. Histological section of Sacrocaudalis dorsalis medialis of a highly marbled, high Wagyu content (75%) heifer M621 (wy75 dx25). Field selected to show eosinophilic rounded fibers of variable size, with abundant perimysial connective tissue in their proximity. Formalin-fixed H & E, MSA MB 820, DOF 471. CYO lab number Ch18/109Y. See also Figure 2 for macroscopic features such as coarse marbling.

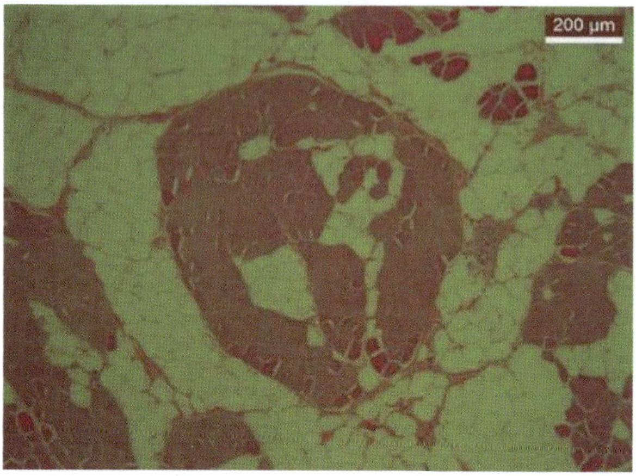

Figure 7. Histological section of Sacrocaudalis dorsalis medialis of a highly marbled, high Wagyu content steer (88%) (wy63 ak25 dx13), showing aggressive adipose invasion, with abundant perimysial connective tissue and the generation of island-like areas of fibers with evident architectural changes including shrinkage of fibers as the front advances. Formalin-fixed H & E, MSA MB 1100, DOF 471. CYO lab number Ch18/110G. See also Figures 1, 4, and 5.

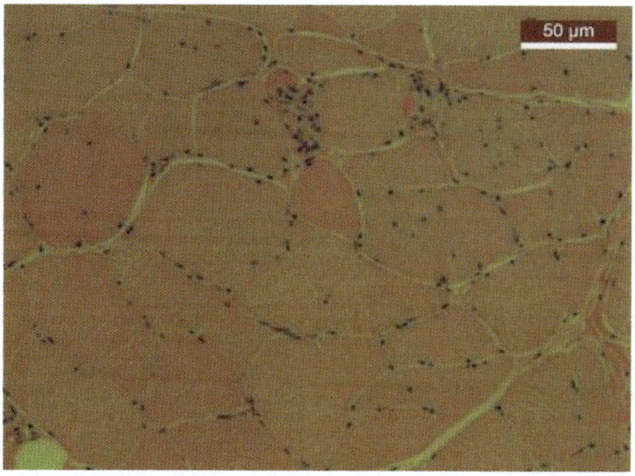

Figure 8. Histological section of Sacrocaudalis dorsalis medialis of a highly marbled, high Wagyu content steer (63%), M129 (wy63 dx13). Higher power selected to illustrate variability of fiber size, affinity for eosin, and the presence of intracytoplasmatic and interstitial nuclei. Formalin-fixed H & E, MSA MB 880, DOF 481. CYO lab number Ch18/135Z.

In some fields, there are collections of nuclei including intra-cytoplasmic (Figure 8).

These observations have led us to the conclusion that the extent and type of marbling is a function of the aggressive extension of the advancing adipocytes with secondary loss of myocytes.

Some forms of human dystrophy have very similar histopathology, for example, congenital myopathies as illustrated by Dubowitz et al. [15] and reproduced here in Figure 9.

As in human dystrophies, there can be different degrees depending upon the muscle group and the field selected. Here, we focus on Sacrocaudalis dorsalis medialis, because it is con-

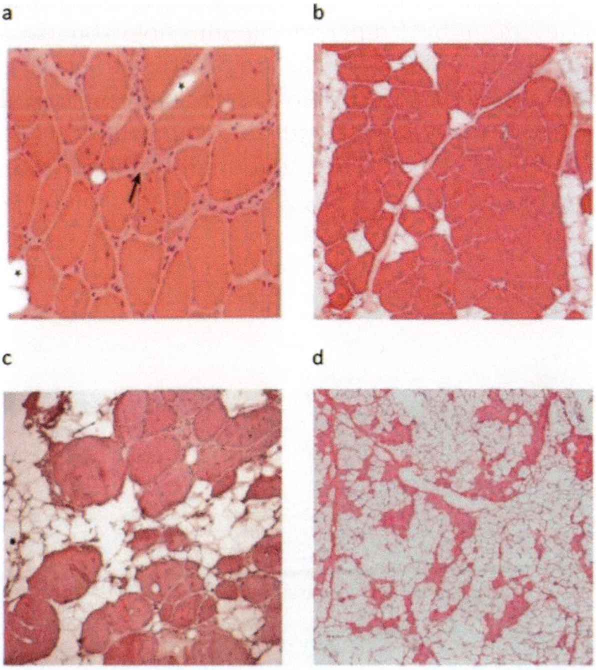

Figure 9. Examples of adipocyte intrusion in human muscular dystrophy. (a) Case of limb-girdle muscular dystrophy showing most fibers surrounded by endomysial connective tissue with some adipocytes (*) ([15], Figure 11.4b). (b) From the deltoid muscle of a patient with ophthalmoplegia associated with a MYH2 mutation showing fatty infiltration, mild fiber atrophy, fibers with internal nuclei, an irregular myofibrillar network, and lobulated fibers ([15], Figure 15.27). (c) From the quadriceps of a patient with facioscapulohumeral dystrophy at 42 years showing pronounced proliferation of connective tissue and fat with a wide variation of muscle cell size and many internal nuclei ([15], Figure 14.1b). (d) Low power view of a biopsy from a case of congenital muscular dystrophy showing only islands of fibers in a vast amount of adipose tissue ([15], Figure 4.30)..

venient to biopsy, whereas the loin can only be accessed readily post-mortem.

Accordingly, it will be possible to undertake detailed time course studies so as to monitor sequential changes and eventually responses to therapy. Future studies should also address bovine steatosis. The pathology [16, 17] is different from marbling. Adipocytes occur within rather than around fascicles (Figure 10) suggesting that the process may be a function of differentiation of stem cells, rather than invasion [1].

7. Conclusion

In spite of similarities in pathology and genomics, there is more to learn before precise translation is possible. However, there are strong indications that such approaches could have important implications for human dystrophies and other muscle diseases. Moreover, a better understanding of the control factors and signals responsible for determining the relative proportions of muscle and adipose tissue in bovine muscles, and how they are coordinated, is fundamental and will be crucial to understanding more fully the significance of adipose tissue replacement in human dystrophies and to developing new therapeutic strategies for these diseases.

Acknowledgments

This research was supported by the CY O'Connor ERADE Village Foundation as publication number MS1803. The authors acknowledge the earlier contributions of J F Williamson

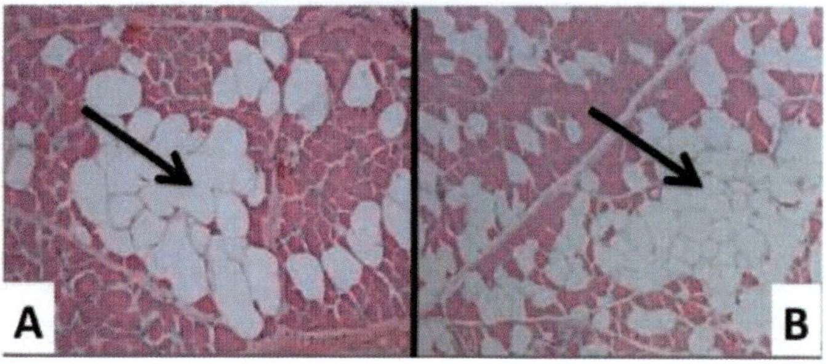

Figure 10. Muscle samples taken from carcasses where steatosis was observed macroscopically at slaughter. Fat infiltration occurs within the muscle fascicle, there are few adipocytes within the perimysium. Used with permission from [17]..

and would like to thank JR Dawkins and Melaleuka Stud for access to the cattle used in this study.

Conflict of interest

Collectively, the authors associated with the CY O'Connor ERADE Village Foundation have an interest in the work described in this manuscript as it forms part of the foundation's intellectual property.

References

[1] Harper GS, Pethick DW. How might marbling begin? Australian Journal of Experimental Agriculture. 2004;**44**:653-662

[2] Tan P, Allen JG, Wilton SD, et al. A splice-site mutation causing ovine McArdle's disease. Neuromuscular Disorders. 1997;**7**:336-342

[3] Ferreiro A, Ceuterick-De Groote C, Marks JJ, et al. Desmin-related myopathy with Mallory body-like inclusions is caused by mutations of the Selenoprotein N gene. Annals of Neurology. 2004;**55**:676-686

[4] Kakulas BA. Regeneration of skeletal muscle in the Rottnest quokka. The Australian Journal of Experimental Biology and Medical Science. 1966;**44**:673-688

[5] Williamson JF, Steele EJ, Lester S, et al. Genomic evolution in domestic cattle: Ancestral haplotypes and healthy beef. Genomics. 2011;**97**:304-312

[6] Dawkins RL, Leelayuwat C, Gaudieri S, et al. Genomics of the major histocompatibility complex: Haplotypes, duplication, retroviruses and disease. Immunological Reviews. 1999;**167**:275-304

[7] Aly TA, Eller E, Ide A, et al. Multi-SNP analysis of MHC region: Remarkable conservation of HLAA1-B8-DR3 haplotype. Diabetes. 2006;**55**:1265-1269

[8] Lloyd SS, Steele EJ, Dawkins RL. Analysis of haplotype sequences. In: Kulski JK, editor. Next Generation Sequencing-Advances, Applications and Challenges. Rijeka, Croatia: InTech; 2016. pp. 345-368

[9] Traherne JA, Horton R, Roberts AN, et al. Genetic analysis of completely sequenced disease-associated MHC haplotypes identifies shuffling of segments in recent human history. PLoS Genetics. 2006;**2**:81-92

[10] Alper CA, Larsen CE, Dubey DP, et al. The haplotype structure of the human major histocompatibility complex. Human Immunology. 2006;**67**:73-84

[11] Dawkins RL, Willamson JF, Lester S, et al. Mutation versus polymorphism in evolution. Genomics. 2013;**101**:211-212

[12] Lloyd SS, Valenzuela JL, Steele EJ, et al. Genetics of marbling in Wagyu revealed by the melting temperature of intramuscular and subcutaneous lipids. International Journal of Food Science. 2017; Article ID 3948408, 6 pages

[13] Lloyd SS, Steele EJ, Valenzuela JL, et al. Haplotypes for type, degree and rate of marbling in cattle are syntenic with human muscular dystrophy. International Journal of Genomics. 2017;**2017**. Article ID 6532837, 14 pages

[14] Valenzuela JL, Lloyd SS, Rebhan H, et al. Monitoring marbling by histology and melting temperature. Pending Publ

[15] Dubowitz V, Sewry CA, Oldfors A, et al. Muscle Biopsy: A Practical Approach. Philadelphia: Saunders Ltd.,2013

[16] Peletto S, Strillacci MG, Capucchio MT, et al. Genetic basis of Lipomatous myopathy in Piedmontese beef cattle. Livestock Science. 2017;**206**:9-16

[17] Biasibetti E, Amedeo S, Brugiapaglia A, et al. Lipomatous muscular dystrophy' of Piedmontese cattle. Animal. 2012;**6**:1839-1847

[18] Tajsharghi H, Hammans S, Lindberg

C, et al. Recessive myosin myopathy with external ophthalmoplegia associated with MYH2 mutations. European Journal of Human Genetics. 2014;**22**:801-808

[19] Lim KS, Lee SH, Lee EA, et al. Effects of intergenic single nucleotide polymorphisms in the fast myosin heavy chain cluster on muscle fiber characteristics and meat quality in Berkshire pigs. Meat Science. Epub ahead of print 2015. DOI: 10.1016/j.meatsci.2015.07.025.

[20] Nobbio L, Visigalli D, Radice D, et al. PMP22 messenger RNA levels in skin biopsies: Testing the effectiveness of a Charcot-Marie-Tooth 1A biomarker. Brain 2014;**137**:1614-1620

[21] Iwata Y, Katanosaka Y, Arai Y, et al. Dominant-negative inhibition of Ca2+ influx via TRPV2 ameliorates muscular dystrophy in animal models. Hum Mol Genet 2009;**18**:824-834

[22] Lloyd DJ, Trembath RC, Shackleton S. A novel interaction between lamin A and SREBP1: implications for partial lipodystrophy and other laminopathies. Hum Mol Genet 2002;**11**:769-778

[23] Hoashi S, Ashida N, Ohsaki H, et al. Genotype of bovine sterol regulatory element binding protein-1 (SREBP-1) is associated with fatty acid composition in Japanese Black cattle. Mamm Genome 2007;**18**:880-886

[24] Surks HK, Riddick N, Ohtani K-I. M-RIP Targets Myosin Phosphatase to Stress Fibers to Regulate Myosin Light Chain Phosphorylation in Vascular Smooth Muscle Cells* Journal of Biological Chemistry. Epub ahead of print 2005. DOI: 10.1074/jbc.M506863200

[25] Dawkins RL, Millman JA, Willamson JF, et al. US9181585B2.pdf. US 9,181,585 B2, United States of America, 2015

[26] Trabelsi M, Kavian N, Daoud F, et al. Revised spectrum of mutations in sarcoglycanopathies. Eur J Hum Genet 2008;**16**:793-803

[27] Moreira ES, Wiltshire TJ, Faulkner G, et al. Limb-girdle muscular dystrophy type 2G is caused by mutations in the gene encoding the sarcomeric protein telethonin. Nat Genet 2000;**24**:163-166

[28] Cheong HS, Yoon D, Kim LH, et al. Titin-cap (TCAP) polymorphisms associated with marbling score of beef. Meat Science. 2007;**77**:257-263

[29] Hayashi YK, Matsuda C, Ogawa M, et al. Human PTRF mutations cause secondary deficiency of caveolins resulting in muscular dystrophy with generalized lipodystrophy. J Clin Invest 2009;**119**:2623-2633

[30] Grumati P, Coletto L, Sabatelli P, et al. Autophagy is defective in collagen VI muscular dystrophies, and its reactivation rescues myofiber degeneration. Nature Medicine 2010;**16**:1313-1320

[31] García-Macia M, Sierra V, Palanca A, et al. Autophagy during beef aging. Autophagy. Epub ahead of print 2014. DOI: 10.4161/auto.26659

[32] Ardiyanti A, Oki Y, Suda Y, et al. Effects of GH gene polymorphism and sex on carcass traits and fatty acid compositions in Japanese Black cattle. Journal of Animal Science. 2009;**80**:62-69

[33] Bhuiyan MSA, Kim YK, Kim HJ, et al. Genome-wide association study and prediction of genomic breeding values for fatty-acid composition in Korean Hanwoo cattle using a highdensity single-nucleotide polymorphism array1. Journal of Animal Science. 2018;**96**:4063-4075

[34] Uemoto Y, Abe T, Tameoka N, et al. Whole-genome association study for fatty acid composition of oleic acid in Japanese Black cattle. Anim Genet 2011;**42**:141-148

[35] Schuelke M, Wagner KR, Stolz LE, et al. Myostatin Mutation Associated with Gross Muscle Hypertrophy in a Child. The New England Journal of Medicine. 2004;**350**:2682-2688

[36] Wiener P, Woolliams JA, Frank-Lawale A, et al. The effects of a mutation in the myostatin gene on meat and carcass quality. Meat Science. Epub ahead of print 2009. DOI: 10.1016/j.meatsci.2009.04.010

[37] Barendse W, Harrison BE, Bunch RJ, et al. Variation at the Calpain 3 gene is associated with meat tenderness in zebu and composite breeds of cattle. BMC

Genetics. Epub ahead of print 2008. DOI: 10.1186/1471-2156-9-41

[38] Casas E, White SN, Riley DG, et al. Assessment of single nucleotide polymorphisms in genes residing on chromosomes 14 and 29 for association with carcass composition traits in Bos indicus cattle. Journal of Animal Science. 2005;83:13-19

[39] Adoligbe CLZ, Farougou S. Functional analysis and association studies of bovine MYOT gene with meat quality. Journal of Animal Science. 2016;**94**:59-60

* * *

Bilateral Amplification of Complementary Duplicons (BACD) identifies local varieties of grasses and their mixtures in pasture: evidence for retrotransposons.

Sally S Lloyd, Anthony J Lloyd, Roger L Dawkins*

Running title: BACD identifies local varieties of grasses

MS 1902 Kikuyu 2019-09-12 submitted Molecular Ecology combined.docx printed 10/12/2019

Centre for Innovation in Agriculture, Murdoch University and C Y O'Connor ERADE Village Foundation, North Dandalup 6207, Western Australia, Australia
*corresponding author slloyd@cyo.edu.au

Abstract

The purpose of the present study is to apply a new method to the resolution of a debate based on speculation as to how Kikuyu grass has changed the ecology of pastures in south western Australia and conversely how Kikuyu grass genetics has adapted to local conditions. We demonstrate that there are differences between known varieties but also between the samples which appear to be recent descendants. Further, we show that there are some similarities and differences between the local samples and those from South Australia where the climate and soil types are similar to south Western Australia. Finally, we show a method to identify Kikuyu grass, clover and ryegrass in mixed pastures.

Keywords: Kikuyu grass, adaptation, retrotransposons, pasture

Introduction

Increasingly over recent decades, Kikuyu grass (*Cenchrus clandestinus* previously known as *Pennisetum clandestinum*) has come to dominate traditional pastures on the coastal plain and, so much so, that many local farmers have attempted elimination. However, others have benefited by the upward creep such that sand hills have become productive.

Kikuyu grass pastures have a high potential productivity with up to 30 t DM/ha annual yield reported for irrigated pasture.(García, Islam, Clark, & Martin, 2014) Irrigated Kikuyu grass is most productive during summer and autumn, filling a feed gap when ryegrass based pastures in south-western Australia are unavailable. Concerns from dairy farmers about lower feed quality are being addressed with optimisation of irrigation, fertiliser and grazing management achieving Metabolisable Energy values of 9.5 to 10.2 MJ/kg DM (Hutton, 2019).Projects to improve the feed quality through genetic modification (Lucksett, Kaiser, & Virgona, 1996) or selection have been less successful. Kikuyu grass is an extremely deep rooting perennial pasture with roots down to 2m. (Nie et al., 2008) Root density of >6500 /m2 in the sub soil to 1m and 750 /m2 in the deep sub soil to 2m increases soil organic matter and allows kikuyu access to the surface aquifer.

Kikuyu Grass is originally a forest margin plant originating from the highlands of eastern and central Africa. Its natural habitat is at elevations between 1950 and 2700 m and average annual rainfall between 1000 and 1600 mm. Typically, the soils in the natural range are deep lateritic red loams of volcanic origin. (Mears, 1970).

A review of archival records of importations of Kikuyu grass into Australia (Morris, 2009) indicates there were a relatively small number (perhaps as few as 5 or 6 separate lines) of importations from 1918 through to the 1930s from which farmers along the East, South and South-West coastal regions of Australia were enthusiastically encouraged by state authorities to plant for pasture production.

Some strains of Kikuyu grass are male sterile and setting of seed was not observed until the 1930s (Morris, 2009). There are practical difficulties in collecting seed and this was not practical on a commercial basis until after 1970.(Mears, 1970) As a consequence, the primary method of propagation until after 1970 was vegetative with stolons obtained initially from state officials and subsequently from neighbouring farmers.(Cullity, 1948)

From 1958, trials of importations from Kenya have resulted in the release of a number of named varieties, of which "Whittet" in 1970 has been the most successful with seed commercially available.

By 1970, Kikuyu grass pastures originating from the introductions from 1918 to the 1930s were successfully established in Australia, across a diverse set of agricultural environments, many quite different from its natural range. Successful adaptation by a species from such a narrow genetic base, with limited sexual reproduction, is by no means rare but sometimes regarded as a paradox (Stapley, Santure, & Dennis, 2015).

At issue, is the degree to which there has been rapid local genetic adaptation. The method chosen to measure the degree of change was developed to distinguish between vertebrate species and their hybrids. Bilateral Amplification of Complementary Duplicons (BACD) utilises a single primer which targets retroviral like elements thought to be important in the process of speciation. The method identifies quantitative differences between horses, mules and donkeys as examples. Surprisingly, there are also differences between invertebrates and between plants. Here we ask whether BACD can resolve the debate over the degree of local adaptation of Kikuyu grass.

We demonstrate that there are differences between known varieties but also between the samples which appear to be recent descendants. Further, we show that there are some similarities and differences between the local samples and those from a South Australia where the climate and soil types are similar to south western Australia. Finally, BACD is able to identify Kikuyu grass, clover and ryegrass in mixed pastures.

The research project's objective is to identify Kikuyu grass strains which were adapted to a classic Mediterranean climate (hot dry summers) and sandy, low nutrient soils. Collections focussed on such pastures in southern and south western Australia which were established prior to 1970 or derived from such sources.

Materials and Methods

Sample collection and DNA extraction.

Kikuyu plants were collected from pasture, garden, park and roadside locations.

Single species samples of leaf and stalk were collected from local pastures for Kikuyu grass, balansa clover and ryegrass (variety Abundant). These samples were air dried at 40degrees for 2hrs and then ground using a CT 293 Cyclotec™ mill (Foss) with a 1mm screen. This is the same procedure used to prepare pasture samples for NIR feed quality tests. DNA was extracted from 200mg of the dry powder using a DNeasy plant mini kit (Qiagen).

The DNA concentration was measured spectrophotometrically (260nm absorption ND-100 Nanodrop) and dilutions prepared at 5ng/ul.

Two species mixtures of Kikuyu grass/ryegrass and Kikuyu grass/clover were prepared from these dilutions at 4:1,1:1 and 1:4 ratios. Three species mixtures of ryegrass, clover and Kikuyu grass were prepared from the extracted DNA at 3:6:11 ratio (by volume). Three species mixtures of ryegrass, clover and Kikuyu grass were also prepared from the powdered dry sample at 3:6:11 ratio (by dry weight), prior to DNA extraction.

BACD PCR reaction

The BACD test was developed as a method of species identification and is described in more detail in (Laird et al., 2006).
10ul reactions with PCR kit: Fisher Biotech Taq F1 DNA Polymerase, 5uM Primer: 5′- ATGAGCTTGTCTACACCT-3′ and 1ng/ul DNA sample.
PCR cycling conditions
95°C x 2min activation, 40 cycles of (94°Cx30s denature, 43°C x 30s annealing, 72°Cx1min extension) with a final 72°Cx5min extension.

Capillary Electrophoresis:

Qiaxcel (Qiagen) with a High Resolution cartridge, method OH800 and 15-1kb alignment marker. Band intensity for the comparison bands was tabulated on a scale of 1-9 using the system first described in (Dawkins et al., 1989).

Sequencing:

BACD PCR reaction was performed for 5 samples with positive and negative examples of each polymorphic band. The products were separated on a 2% agarose gel (for 24 hrs at E=2V/cm). Bands were cut out of gel, DNA purified with Wizard Plus SV Minipreps (Promega). The presence of the correct product was checked by capillary electrophoresis. In several cases more than one band was present in the extraction. For this reason, because more than one sequence was expected in the high concentration bands, the selected products were cloned into competent E coli cells using the TOPO TA Cloning Kit (Invitrogen). A number of bacterial colonies were chosen for amplification and cloning, depending on the intensity of the extracted bands so as to ensure at least one reaction would contain the desired product. The products were sequenced
The resulting sequences were compared to each other using Gepard and matched against Retrotransposon databases from

all plants using CENSOR.(Jurka, Klonowski, Dagman, & Pelton, 1996)

Results

Detection of three species in mixed pastures

Samples of ryegrass, clover and Kikuyu grass gave distinctly different profiles when tested using the BACD primers. The amplicon lengths and intensities are characteristic at a species level. Different varieties of ryegrass and Kikuyu grass gave similar, but not identical profiles. Typical profiles are shown in Figure 1, with band lengths of some species-specific amplicons identified. We sequenced several amplicons from the 730bp bands from ryegrass and clover. Each band was made up of several sequences, with some showing no similarity other than the length and priming site. We did not find any sequence from the ryegrass 730bp band that was similar to sequences from the clover 730bp band.

The intensity of the band patterns were tabulated using an in-house scheme (Dawkins et al., 1989) which permits a degree of standardisation from run to run and from sample to sample and allows the development of a database for detailed analysis. In Figure 2 we show that the intensity of species specific bands in samples containing a mixture of pastures varied according to the relative amounts of DNA from each species.

BACD Identifies genetic variation between commercial Kikuyu grass varieties and naturalized specimens

Three bands at 184bp, 386bp and 509bp showed variation among the samples of 5 different commercial varieties tested (1 pasture and 4 turf). The results are shown in Table 1.

There were an additional two bands (432bp and 468bp) that showed variation within the 123 samples collected from roadsides, gardens and established pastures. The 432bp band was present in all of the commercial samples but absent in 20% of the naturalised samples. The 468bp band was present in 61% of these samples, but in none of the commercial varieties tested (see Table 2). This contrast between the commercial samples and the majority of the naturalized samples suggests either that the naturalized population draws more substantially from the early, non seed-producing imports or that it is connected to the local ecology driving adaptation. A role for retrotransposons is suggested.

The BACD results divide the collected samples into 19 groups of similar genetics (Sup Fig 1). Nearly half of the collected samples are within one BACD defined group. Using this initial screening test will improve the efficiency of subsequent phenotype selection by maximizing the initial genetic variation within a smaller sample set.

Sequencing of informative products confirms the presence of indels and reveals a diversity of retrotransposons.

We used Sanger sequencing of the amplicons from Kikuyu grass to identify the type of genetic variations detected between Kikuyu grass varieties. Dotplot comparisons using Gepard (Krumsiek, Arnold, & Rattei, 2007) revealed that the 386bp and 509bp amplicons were very similar to each other, with the difference in length almost entirely due to one indel of 120bp (See Figure 3). There was very little similarity between any of the other amplicon sequences of different lengths.

All of the amplicons were compared against all plant retrotransposons submitted to the retrotransposon database "Repbase".(Bao, Kojima, & Kohany, 2015) The genome of Kikuyu grass has not been substantially sequenced and no retrotransposons from it are included in the database, nor any from the same genus (*Cenchrus* or *Pennisetum*) so exact matches were not expected. The retrotransposons that best match each amplicon are shown in Table 2. More than 70% of the product sequence could be matched to retrotransposons on the database, with only one amplicon not containing any known retrotransposon. The matched retrotransposons came from three species of grasses: Sorghum (*Sorghum bicolor*), Maize (*Zea mays*) and foxtail millet (*Setaria italica*). These three species are, like Kikuyu grass, C4 grasses. The sequence similarity ranged from 63% to 78%.

An alignment of the 509bp and 386bp amplicons with the Copia-69_SB-I retrotransposon is shown in Fig 4. The 509bp amplicons aligns to the retrotransposon across the full length of the indel, while the 386bp is missing a portion of this retrotransposon, but matches with reasonable similarity on either side.

Discussion

This study has shown similarities between varieties in 3 widely separated regions with similar soils and climate. Further sampling is required to establish whether these are soil and climate specific in relation to different regions, but the current methods and database appear appropriate and therefore justify characterisation of the defining amplicons and their relevance to adaptation in differing environments. An important by-product of the present study is our demonstration that an extremely simple and cheap method can monitor the species composition of mixed pastures. We have also shown that the BACD test can be used to confirm the variety of Kikuyu grass sold.

Acknowledgements

We would like to thank Joanne Rollinson and Matthew Nippierd for their work on this project and to Ray Candy and Adrian Pitsikas for providing samples and background. This is publication 1902 of the CY O'Connor ERADE Village Foundation supported by funding from a Regional Grant Scheme administered by the Peel Development Commission of Western Australia.

Data Accessibility

DNA sequences and sample locations will be made available in supplementary data files.

References

Bao, W., Kojima, K. K., & Kohany, O. (2015). Repbase Update, a database of repetitive elements in eukaryotic genomes. *Mobile DNA*, *6*(1), 4–9. doi: 10.1186/s13100-015-0041-9

Cullity, M. (1948). Kikuyu grass. *Journal of the Department of Agriculture of Western Australia*, *25*, 185–198.

Dawkins, R. L., Leaver, A., Cameron, P. U., Martin, E., Kay, P. H., & Christiansen, F. T. (1989). Some disease-associated ancestral haplotypes carry a polymorphism of TNF. *Human Immunology*, *26*(2), 91–97. doi: 10.1016/0198-8859(89)90094-3

García, S. C., Islam, M. R., Clark, C. E. F., & Martin, P. M. (2014). Kikuyu-based pasture for dairy production: a review. *Crop and Pasture Science*, *65*(8), 787. doi:

10.1071/cp13414

Hutton, P. (2019, March). Kikuyu as an irrigated summer pasture. *Feed Trough.* Retrieved from https://www.dairyaustralia.com.au/publications/feed-trough?id=590916583A964C77A374A5E91854BA3C

Jurka, J., Klonowski, P., Dagman, V., & Pelton, P. (1996). CENSOR- a program identification and elimination of repetitive elements from DNA sequences. *Comp Chem, 20*(20), 119–121.

Krumsiek, J., Arnold, R., & Rattei, T. (2007). Gepard: A rapid and sensitive tool for creating dotplots on genome scale. *Bioinformatics, 23*(8), 1026–1028. doi: 10.1093/bioinformatics/btm039

Laird, R., Gaudieri, S., Berry, J., Williamson, J., Yang, J.-S., & Dawkins, R. (2006). Vertebrate Species profiling in one step using a single primer. *Forensic Science Medicine and Pathology*, *2*(3), 165–172. doi: 10.1385/Forensic

Lucksett, D., Kaiser, A., & Virgona, J. (1996). *Innovative breeding of kikuyu cultivators to increase milk production.* Retrieved from https://www.mla.com.au/research-and-development/search-rd-reports/final-report-details/Productivity-On-Farm/Innovative-breeding-of-high-digestibility-kikuyu-cultivators-to-increase-milk-production/1772#

Mears, P. T. (1970). Kikuyu as a pasture grass - a review. *Tropical Grasslands*, *4*(2), 139.

Morris, B. (2009). *Variation and Breeding of Kikuyu Grass (Pennisetum clandestinum).* University of Sydney.

Nie, Z. N., Miller, S., Moore, G. A., Hackney, B. F., Boschma, S. P., Reed, K. F. M., … Dear, B. S. (2008). Field evaluation of perennial grasses and herbs in southern Australia. 2. Persistence, root characteristics and summer activity. *Australian Journal of Experimental Agriculture, 48*(4), 424. doi: 10.1071/ea07136

Stapley, J., Santure, A. W., & Dennis, S. R. (2015). Transposable elements as agents of rapid adaptation may explain the genetic paradox of invasive species. *Molecular Ecology*, *24*, 2241–2252. doi: 10.1111/mec.13089

Figures and Tables

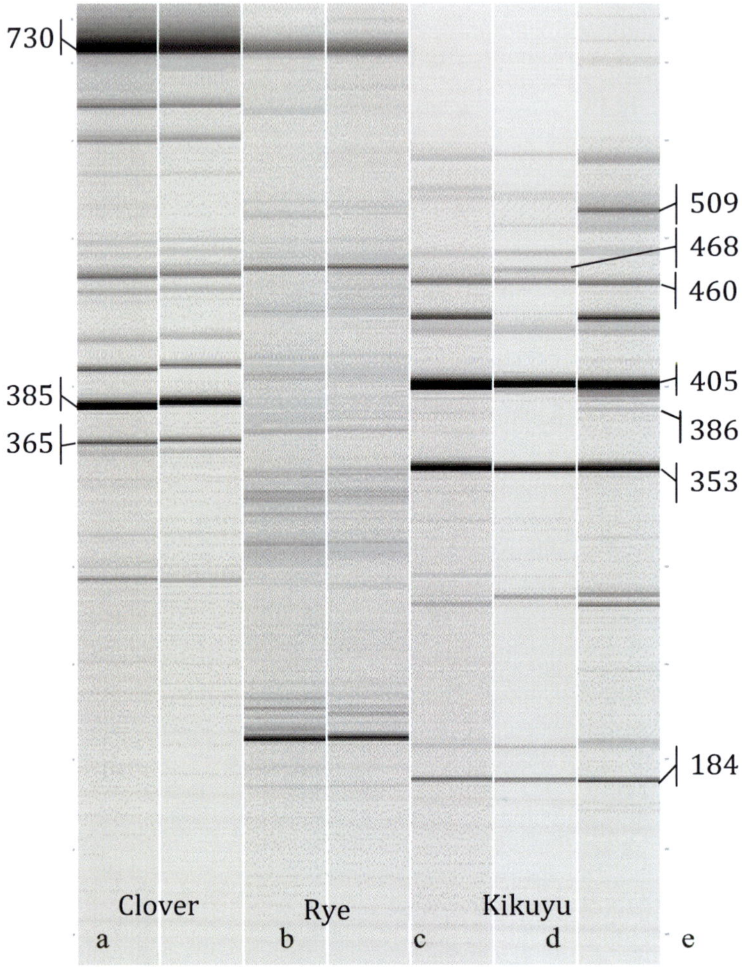

Figure 1: Detection of three species in mixed pastures.

The BACD probe reveals unequivocal qualitative differences between the dominant ryegrass clover and kikuyu species. a,b)Balansa clover (same sample) c)ryegrass "Burst" d) ryegrass "Abundant" e,f,g) kikuyu (3 naturalised specimens).

The separation of bands is sensitive to changes in temperature and concentration (comparison of a and b columns from different CE runs), and the intensity dependent on quality and concentration of sample DNA. The species and variety band patterns were clear and were confirmed by reference samples included with each run. Results were tabulated standardising against these reference samples.

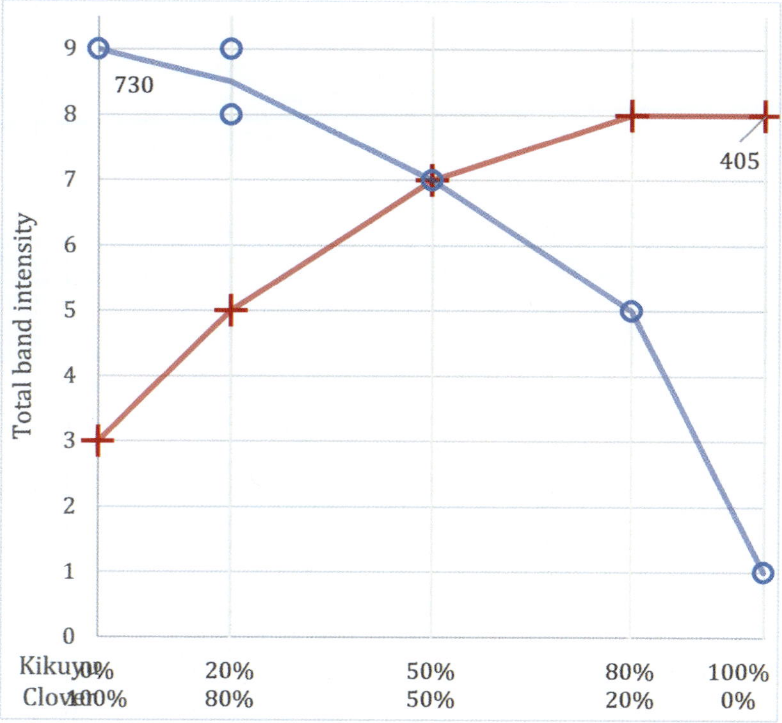

Figure 2: The content of mixed pastures can be defined by quantifying species markers.

The highest intensity band from kikuyu and clover are shown, but other bands changed intensity in a similar manner. The horizontal axis shows the proportion of kikuyu and clover DNA in the mixed sample, while the vertical axis shows the intensity of the band, assessed visually using a logarithmic scale from 1-9 (Dawkins 1989).

Table 1: BACD probe reveals quantitative differences between recognised varieties of kikuyu

Variety	Intensity of Amplicon		
	184bp	386bp	509bp
Whittet	1	1	5
Regal	6	1	3
Village Green	6	1	1
Kenda	6	3	1
Emerald	6	3	1

Figure 3: Sequencing of informative products confirms the presence of indels

Comparison of sequence for the 386bp and 509bp products show that they are very similar except for a 120bp indel(dotplot using Gepard)

Table 2: Differences also reveal a diversity of retrotransposons

Frequency in samples		amplicon length	Matching Retrotransposon†	Species of retrotransposon	Proportion of amplicon	Sequence similarity
naturalised	commercial					
90%	86%	184	Gypsy-88_ZM-I	Maize	85%	78%
100%	100%	353	none identified		0%	
18%	43%	386	Copia-69_SB-I/ Copia-39_Sit-I	Sorghum/ Foxtail millet	94%	76%, 75%
100%	100%	405	Gypsy-120_SB-I	Sorghum	76%	63%
80%	100%	432	Gypsy-124N_SBi-LTR	Sorghum	40%	75%
100%	100%	~460		Not sequenced		
62%	0%	~468		Not sequenced		
13%	43%	509	Copia-69_SB-I	Sorghum	96%	77%

†Retrotransposons identified using Censor matched against database of all retrotransposons identified in plants.

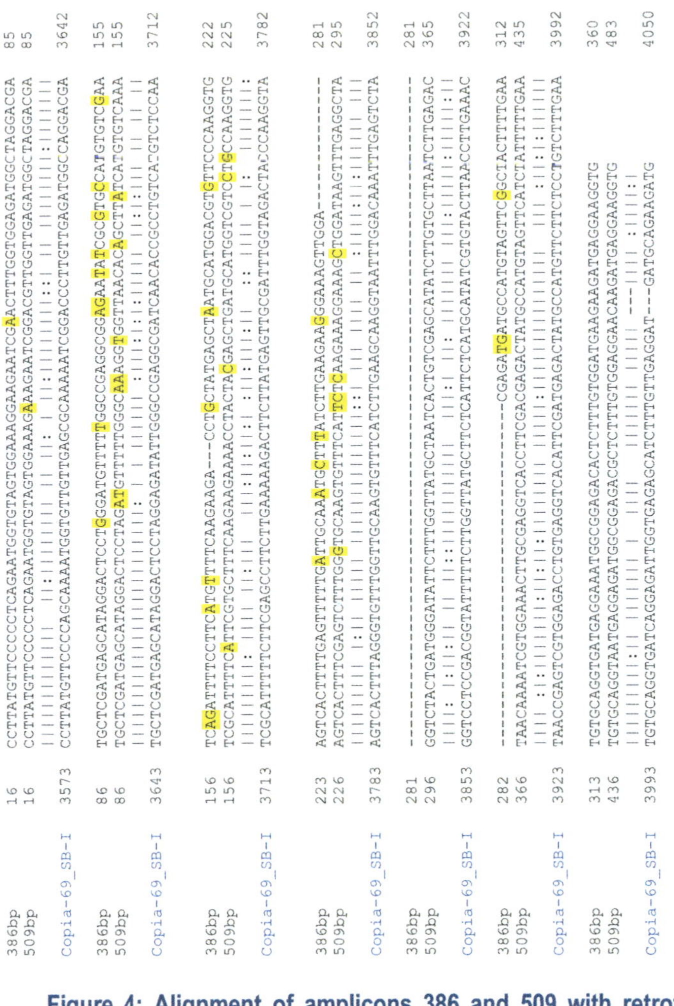

Figure 4: Alignment of amplicons 386 and 509 with retrotransposon Copia-69_SB-I.

Alignment between 509bp amplicon and Copia-69_SB-I retrotransposon produced by CENSOR. Yellow shading highlights where the two amplicon sequences are different, and which differs from the retrotransposon.

Supplementary table 1: Additional polymorphism not in commercial varieties is revealed in collected ecotypes

Group	Band strength					No. samples				
	184	386	509	432	468	Total	S.A.	Peel	Albany	Commercial
7b	1	1	4-5	5-6	1	3		1		1a
7a	1	1	1	6	1	1				
8a	1	3	1	6	1	1	1			
8b	1	4	5	6	1	1			1	
9b	5-6	1	3-4	5-6	1	4		1	2	1b
9a	3-7	1	1	3-7	1	15		9	3	2c
10b	5-6	4-6	4-5	4-6	1	2		1	1	
10a	5-6	3-5	1	5-7	1	11	1	6		2 d,e
13	1	1	1	3-7	4-5	3		2	1	
11a	4-7	1	1	4-6	3-6	57	3	27	10	
11b	5-6	1	3-5	6-7	4-5	3	1	1		
12a	7	4	1	6	5	1				
12b	5-7	3	3-5	6	4-5	2		1	1	
6	1	1	1	1	1	2		1		
5	1	3	4-5	1	1	2				
4	5-6	1	1	1	1	12		5	2	
1	1	1	1	1	4-6	1		1		
3	5-6	1	1	1	5	4		2	2	
2	5	3	1	1	3-6	4	1			

a) Whittet, b) Regal c) Village Green d) Kenda e) Emerald

Features

Beware of blaming livestock for human extravagance: Accept your accumulated ancestry and only disconnect with caution.

RL Dawkins

There seems to be a fashion for diverting blame from the human consumer and polluter by implicating the very animals which have allowed humans to flourish until they wantonly overpopulate the world. The cow is now cast as the villain whereas she was venerated by our forebears. Rightly so, since she has fostered human development allowing children to survive a perilous childhood, develop the brains of intelligent adults and adapt to the continuing use of dairy products.

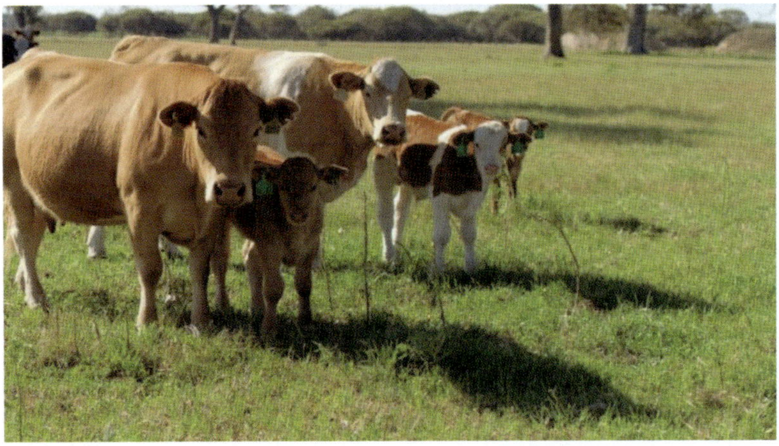

The cow is the "wet-nurse of... civilisation", "the mother of immunisation" and "man's better friend".

There have been cultural differences in the nature of the relationship between humans and cattle or sheep, goats, camels, horses and other lactating breeds, suggesting that the benefits of coexistence with other mammals were widely appreciated. Although most attention is given to the 'fertile crescent' as the cradle of agriculture, domestication, clustering and then civilisation, it is certain that similar processes were occurring wherever conditions allowed. Time-frames varied but as a generalisation it is safe to assume that humans have benefitted from other mammals for thousands of years and therefore hundreds or even thousands of generations. From an evolutionary perspective, much can happen in even a few generations exposed to changes in food, drink, culture, poisons, climate and to cohabitation with animals and their microbes. Favourable DNA sequences were selected by changing environments and have been conserved. We are therefore the fortunate survivors of all these challenges. It is simply not possible to reverse the adaptive changes now encoded in DNA. Therefore, it is unknown what may happen if we are persuaded to inflict new variations to past experience. There are no shortages of advocates for change for whatever reason, but rarely does this advice come with some understanding of the potential implications. Fashions, religious zeal and passions can be dangerous and increasingly so in the current era of social media.

It is often not appreciated how the cow has contributed in so many ways. Milk is just one gift but perhaps the most important. In addition to its nutritional value, especially for survival and brain development in childhood, milk provided a degree of passive immunity and therefore protection from shared microbes. Milk products which could be stored safely, such as cheese, were crucial in winter and allowed worldwide exploration of better environments, as exemplified by the Dutch after developing successful pastures and dairies.

Meat was also crucial to hunter gatherers and most cultures subsequently. So too were cattle used for energy, including warmth and transport. Hides and horns had many uses and fertiliser is thought to have been a critical facilitator of crops. In addition to these obvious contributions, cattle and other ruminants convert combustible forage such as cellulose into useful food - which humans cannot do. Further, they can drink filthy water which would be fatal for humans but yields sanitised milk.

Less appreciated is the role of cattle in controlling infectious disease such as human smallpox. Devastating epidemics were controlled by exposure to cow pox since the relevant virus is sufficiently similar to confer immunity in humans. There are other examples of beneficial exposure to infections carried by domesticated livestock but also warnings as, for example, in the case of TB and BSE. A principle emerges. Managed relationships with other mammals are beneficial but cannibalism is patently dangerous. Take Kuru as an example of the importance of understanding transmissible agents. Health regulations for eating meat or drinking milk are well understood, sensible and widely practised although some activists cannot be convinced of pasteurisation and vaccination. Worse still are the persistent claims that (red) meat causes cancer. There are so many concomitant factors to blame, such as environmental pollution, over processing, untested additives, transfats, creative cooking etc and so many causes of cancer, it is difficult to understand why this claim receives focus unless there are ulterior motives such as the promotion of other foods or subjective beliefs.

The broader issue of whether it is now morally "unacceptable" to eat meat and cheese or to drink milk might be judged against the need to feed the world with food which has been tested over generations and found to be safe. Activism has generated hostility towards the farmers who provide that food. Animal welfare should not be the issue since farmers are much better practitioners than activists. Slaughter may be offensive to those who prefer animals to die in suffering and senility or at the mercy of predators. Suppose the current arrangements were suspended and livestock were left to die in the field in the absence of even minimal care and euthanasia. Then predators would flourish and their diseases would be undetected and eventually rampant. Livestock might prefer "happy life, happy death" with effective control of contagious disease. Humans may come to expect something similar for themselves.

It should also be understood that combustible waste from unmanaged vegetation contributes CO_2 to the atmosphere whilst regrowth of continually grazed perennial pastures actually extracts CO_2 and improves the soil. Consider also the implications of blaming livestock for methane. The effects are short lived and, in any event, methane is also produced by growing rice crops. By way of summary, it is time for agriculture to respond to negative statements with convincing arguments. The following quotes provide some sources.

Daily, ARS focuses on solutions to agricultural problems affecting America. Each dollar invested in agricultural research results in $20 of economic impact.

The Agricultural Research Service (U.S. Department of Agriculture's in-house research agency).

"Among the results to emerge thus far: ... beef cattle production accounted for 3.3 percent of all U.S. GHG emissions (By comparison, transportation and electricity generation together made up 56 percent of the total in 2016 and agriculture in general 9 percent). Fossil energy (for example, fuel) use in cattle production accounted for less than 1 percent of the total consumed nationally. Cattle only consumed 2.6 pounds of grain per pound of beef cut weight (or, butchered carcass weight), which was comparable to pork and poultry."

A brief history of meat in the human diet and current health implications. Neil J. Mann

In Elsevier; Meat Science, Vol 144, Oct 2018, pp 169-179

Abstract "Anthropological investigations have confirmed many times over, through multiple fields of research the critical role of consumption of animal source foods (ASF) including meat in the evolution of our species. As early as four million years ago, our early bipedal hominin ancestors were scavenging ASFs as evidenced by cut marks on animal bone remains, stable isotope composition of these hominin remains and numerous other lines of evidence from physiological and paleo-anthropological domains. This ASF intake marked a transition from a largely forest dwelling frugivorous lifestyle to a more open rangeland existence and resulted in numerous adaptations, including a rapidly increasing brain size and altered gut structure. Details of the various fields of anthropological evidence are discussed, followed by a summary of the health implications of meat consumption in the modern world, including issues around saturated fat and omega-3 fatty acid intake and discussion of the critical nutrients ASFs supply, with particular emphasis on brain function."

Methane Sources – Rice Paddies

GreenHouse Gas Online, All about greenhouse gas science

At between 50 and 100 million tonnes of methane a year, rice agriculture is a big source of atmospheric methane, possibly the biggest of man-made methane sources. The warm, waterlogged soil of rice paddies provides ideal conditions for methanogenesis, and though some of the methane produced is usually oxidized by methanotrophs in the shallow overlying water, the vast majority is released into the atmosphere. ..."

Akaushi will be the breed that contributes - A Cooper

Quality and consistency will continue to be important to beef consumers in the future. Accountability, traceability and healthiness will become increasingly important to beef consumers. There will be continued industry exposure to source verification and certification of husbandry practices with auditing. Consumer premiums will reflect an aggregate of these factors.

As a cattle producer, the goal is to raise beef cattle in extensive operations within a commercial budget yet market on a premium basis. Akaushi will be the breed that contributes greatly. Akaushi are the most biologically efficient cattle in producing beef with elevated levels of marbling above commodity product while being raised in extensive environments.

Commercial cattle producers are receiving and demanding more information when purchasing fullblood/purebred bulls. Stud breeders will continue to demand their breed associations provide scientific selection tools for use in breeding and marketing. Genomics will be the primary focus, but holding generationally proven phenotypic criteria as a priority will be the greatest challenge. *30 October, 2019*

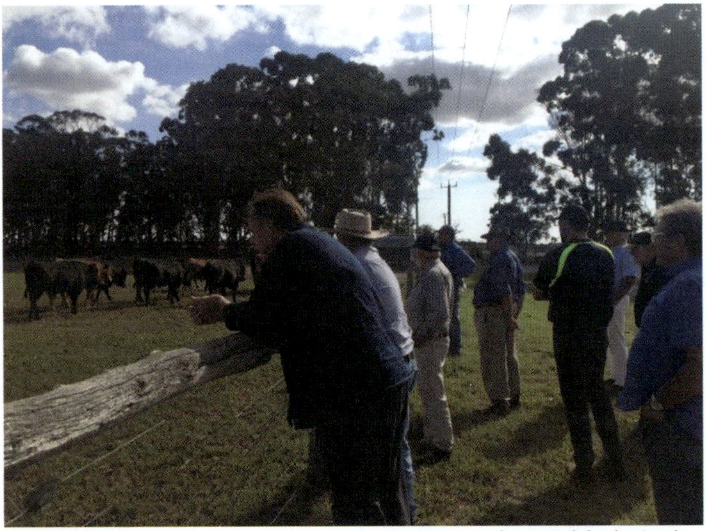

Meeting delegates Inspecting Akaushi and Wagyu cattle at Melaleuka Stud

Kikuyu Improvement Project Report – AJ Lloyd

Supported by the Western Australian Government Royalties for Regions Program and the Peel Development Commission.
September 2019

Contents

1. Background

The Kikuyu Improvement Project is part of the Foundation's scientific research work aimed at improving agricultural productivity and environmental outcomes within the Peel Region.

Kikuyu Grass (*Cenchrus clandestinus,* formerly *Pennisetum clandestinus*) is a summer-growing perennial pasture plant widely used in Australia for a century. It has been important in livestock production (dairy and meat) regions with summer rainfall or availability of irrigation due to its productivity, persistence and hardiness. Within the Peel Region it is commonly used in conjunction with winter growing pasture species.

Kikuyu grass is a forest margin plant originating from the highlands of eastern and central Africa. Its natural habitat is at elevations between 1950 and 2700 m and average annual rainfall between 1000 and 1600 mm. Typically, the soils in Kikuyu's natural range are deep lateritic red loams of volcanic origin.

Kikuyu was initially introduced to the East Coast of Australia from Southern Africa in 1919 and was widely propagated along the east coast of Australia and in South Australia.

By the 1940s, Kikuyu was widespread in coastal districts of south-west Western Australia. Its establishment mirrored that in other parts of Australia, mainly through vegetative propagation although there were some reports of distribution through animal droppings. There is no evidence of independent importation into Western Australia and it is likely that material was sourced from other parts of Australia soon after its introduction.

Although there were a limited number of separate introductions (perhaps as few as five or six lines by the end of the 1930s), there seems not to have been any attempt to distinguish superior cultivars. In the 1960s a further round of controlled introductions were agronomically assessed resulting in the release of a small number of stable, named varieties, of which "Whittet" is the most common.

One of the advantages of the variety "Whittet" is that it seeds prolifically whereas the previous Kikuyu material was either male sterile or seeded sporadically and in modest amounts. "Whittet" seed is commercially available and constitutes virtually all new plantings.

There has been a common misconception that "common" Kikuyu is genetically uniform despite recent published research evidence. There is also local anecdotal evidence that vegetative plantings from locally sourced material produce superior outcomes. It is certainly the case that "common" Kikuyu is established across a very broad range of climate and soil types in Australia.
It is our hypothesis that local adaptation to local deep, sandy, low nutrient soils will result in plants with a with a greater capacity to capture nutrients (phosphorous and nitrogen) and therefore minimize nutrient pollution in adjacent waterways.

The adaptation of a species to a broad range of environmental conditions from a narrow genetic base is not without precedent but is something of a paradox to the conventional approach of population genetics.

The Foundation therefore embarked on a research program to identify the source and level of genetic diversity and test whether any of the identified strains might form the basis of a cultivar adapted to conditions within the Peel Region.

2. Preliminary Work

In 2016, the Foundation undertook a preliminary collection program within the Peel Region to provide a basis for an initial study.

The Foundation had previously developed a laboratory technique (BACD) which reliably identifies and distinguished animal species on the basis of DNA sequences established at the point of speciation (the creation of new species) and subsequently conserved. More recently, the Foundation's researchers had shown that the same technique, when applied to plants, had the capacity to identify and distinguish varieties and show how they are related.

The Foundation's researchers applied the BACD technique to the small number of samples collected at that stage and demonstrated that the technique reliably identified individual strains and distinguished between them.

3. Regional Grant Scheme Grant

The Foundation applied for a Regional Grant Scheme Grant on 23 March 2017, in the amount of $107,500 and was awarded a grant of $105,000 with the grant agreement executed 19 June 2017.

The project was originally planned to complete by 30 June 2018 but was extended to 30 June 2019.

The project objectives were directed to the identification of strains of Kikuyu Grass which were superior to commercially available strains by reason of their adaptation to the conditions of the Peel Region so as to enhance agricultural productivity and environmental effects. Additional objectives were to establish a better method of measuring feed quality, the training of locally based staff in the relevant technologies and to provide a platform for further research into Kikuyu pasture improvement.

4. Collection Program

As referred to above, the collection program commenced in 2016, from samples submitted by local primary producers and from domestic sources. In 2017 the collection program was extended within the Peel Region and throughout the South West of WA including the south coast. Samples were also collected in South Australia near the lower reaches of the Murray, on the basis of similar climate and soil types to those with the Peel region. Additional sample collections continue as results require. The areas of sample collection are set out in Figures 1 and 2.

The original project plan anticipated that samples would be duplicated and grown out in greenhouse facilities at Challenger TAFE at Murdoch. In the event, the Foundation was able to utilise its shadehouse facilities under sprinkler irrigation in North Dandalup for that purpose, saving travelling time and expense. Equipment was obtained from the greenhouse supplies at Murdoch University.

5. Genetic Analysis

As referred to above, the Foundation had previously developed the BACD technique. We postulated the technique has the capacity to identify those DNA sequences which are implicated in the biological mechanisms resulting in the different characteristics of particular varieties or strains.

The BACD technique is well suited to the identification and analysis of a population which shows rapid development of genetic diversity from a small founder population. Such situations are often the initial conditions for speciation events and in the case of new invasive species. The rapid development of genetic diversity is often evidenced by the duplication of sequences from one part of the genome to another part. These sequences are called transposable elements (TE) and in many

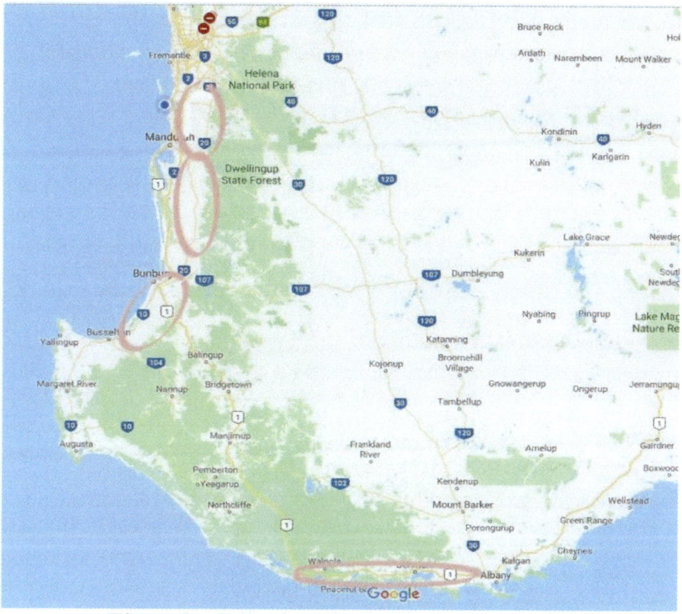

Figure 1: Collection sites in Western Australia

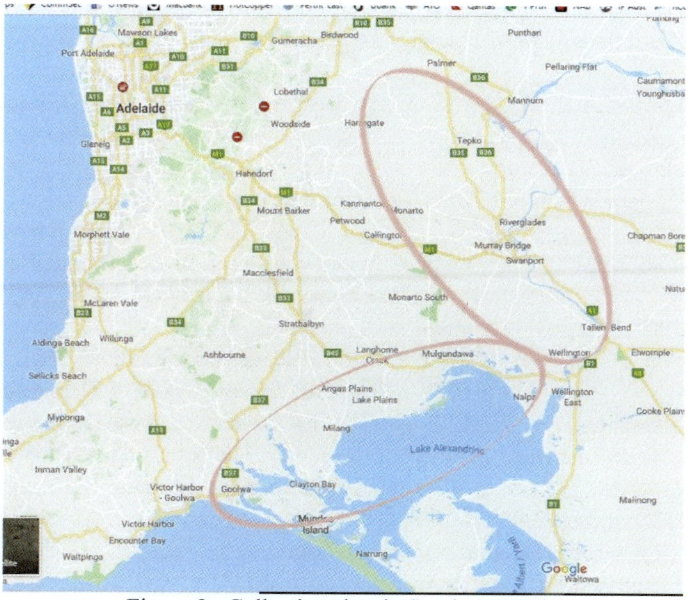

Figure 2: Collection sites in South Australia

cases are the remnants of retroviral infections (retrotransposons) within the host DNA. The BACD test identifies sequences characterised by retrotransposon signatures by extracting sequences of varying lengths (PCR products). By further laboratory procedures, the PCR products are isolated and provide the basis for subsequent DNA sequencing.

DNA was extracted from each of the collected samples and the BACD technique applied. On the basis of the DNA differences established by the BACD technique, the collected samples were allocated into genetically identical or near-identical plants.

PCR products which by their presence or absence (alone or in combination) defined the groups were isolated and sequenced. The sequences demonstrated that variations in product length were in part the result of insertions and deletions within the same sequences.

The sequences were also compared with databases of retrotransposons found in other grass species demonstrating similarity with families of retrotransposons present on those other grasses.

Two PCR products showed particular differences between commercially available varieties. The 432bp product was present in all five commercial varieties but absent in 20% of the naturalised samples, while the 468bp product was absent from all the commercial varieties but present in 61% of the naturalised samples.

The genetic analysis is reported in the annexed paper submitted to a peer-reviewed Journal. The results support our hypothesis of genetic diversity driven by retrotransposon activity within an originally small founder population rapidly expanding mainly through vegetative propagation. It supports the strategy of identifying locally adapted strains from within local populations to isolate superior individual plants for improved productivity.

The results also form a basis as a screening tool to eliminate genetically similar plants from future collection activity.
Those sequences (and the insertion/deletions) will be compared with the results of field trials. This may illuminate the

molecular mechanisms by which different plants (and their groups) perform differently, further opening options for selecting improved strains or using other plant breeding techniques.

6. Field Trials

The 19 groups identified by the BACD analysis referred to above comprised 13 primary groups and 6 secondary groups. Examples of those 13 primary groups, together with three duplicates were propagated in pots, grown out and planted out in a field trial under irrigation, using a duplicated randomised block design.

In autumn 2019, samples were taken and subjected to drying, grinding (at the Foundation's laboratory) and near infra-red spectroscopy (NIRS) (by the CSIRO laboratories) to determine the various components of feed value (protein, digestibility, metabolizable energy etc).

The results show some a small number of samples which promise to be superior cultivars, in terms of feed quality. Interestingly, one of those is from a farm within the Shire of Murray, supporting the initial conjecture that there has been local genetic adaptation to local conditions.
When growing conditions improve in the coming spring/summer it will be possible to assess whether the promising cultivars sustain their superiority over an annual production period and under grazing conditions.

7. Training and Employment

A part of the grant was utilized in recruiting a local (Shire of Serpentine- Jarrahdale) TAFE graduate as a Research Assistant and training that person in genetic laboratory techniques prior to her work on the project.

8. Summary and Conclusions

Kikuyu grass is a valuable pasture plant for the Peel livestock industry. It is part of the Foundation's research program to assist the development of agriculture in the Peel Region. To identify and make available a strain of Kikuyu adapted to local conditions and superior to currently available varieties has the potential to improve agricultural productivity in the region, as well as support environmental objectives

The funding has allowed a comprehensive sample collection program, genetic analysis of the collected samples, and field trials to commence. The genetic analysis supports the hypothesis that, since the introduction of a small founder population into Australia a century ago, Kikuyu grass genetic diversity has been driven by subsequent retrotransposon activity and that superior strains for local conditions are likely to be found within the local population or local populations in similar environments.

The field trials have identified a small number of strains with promise but require further testing to confirm their suitability. The sample collection program has resulted in a diverse library of Kikuyu grass plants which are maintained at the Foundations premises in North Dandalup and will form the basis of further research work.

9. The Future

The Kikuyu Improvement Project is a continuing project for the Foundation. The Foundation will continue with field trials to confirm the suitability of strains which have identified to have promise as a superior variety.

The scope of this part of the Foundation's research did not include a consideration of the role of other pasture varieties within the agricultural system. Local farmers commonly use winter growing species such as ryegrasses and clovers to complement summer-dominant Kikuyu. The interactions between these different species (and the grazing animals) is an aspect which warrants further study.

The BACD technique, originally developed as a method to distinguish animal species has been demonstrated by this study to have a much broader utility. As a further example, the technique was applied to loads of grain dust supplied by CBH free to local farmers as a supplementary animal feed, one load of which was implicated in livestock deaths. The results indicated a non-grain component in the grain dust which warrants further research. It is anticipated that further work will be undertaken to understand the implications in collaboration with CBH.

Kikuyu grass will form a part of a future project to trial grass-fed beef production through irrigated perennial pastures with the aim of displacing grain-based feedlots and therefore reducing adverse environmental and animal welfare effects. The project will also identify the extent to which irrigated perennial pastures increase soil carbon (particularly at depth), reducing nutrient export from farms and be a form of carbon sequestration.

The genetic analysis will continue with the aim of determining the genetic basis of superior adaptations contributing to future screening and breeding programs.

10. Recommendations for further work

A. The established field trial should be continued to confirm superior locally adapted strains and to establish the relevance of the BACD-identified differences.

B. Superior locally adapted strains should be assessed for seed production capacity and, if male sterile, a breeding program adopted to produce a seeding variety while maintaining its superior characteristics.

C. The extent to which superior stains in a monoculture situation, retain that superiority in various pasture mixes.

D. The contribution of summer-irrigated Kikuyu pastures may make to increasing soil carbon (particularly at soil depths up to 2 metres) and sequestration of carbon.

E. The non-grain components of grain-dust residues used as supplementary livestock feed (in collaboration with CBH)

11. Acknowledgments

The Foundation acknowledges the support of the Western Australian government through the Royalty for Regions Program and the Peel Development Commission for their support for this project. The Foundation also acknowledges the support of farmers in the Peel Region for their contributions in relation to samples and field trials.

In The Press

Akaushi genetics to boost beef output

Mal Gill ***Published Farm Weekly, 27 Oct 2018***

FOR a West Texas cattleman out of San Angelo, once exclusively Longhorns territory, Aaron Cooper knows a lot about Japanese cows and bulls. His specialty is the Akaushi breed, which is often referred to as Red Wagyu and is commonly mistaken as simply a colour variation of the Black Wagyu renowned for its fat marbling. His knowledge is not surprising, since Texas is home to the world's largest full-blood Akaushi breeding herd outside of Japan. It is also home to the HeartBrand Beef operation, global leader in Akaushi cattle, genetics and branded beef production. Thanks primarily to HeartBrand's effective marketing, Akaushi as a cattle breed and as a 'brand' of premium beef is more widely recognised by United States consumers than Wagyu, supporters of the Japanese breeds agree. Dr Cooper, who has an animal science degree from Texas A&M University and a Masters degree in animal breeding and genetics from University of Nebraska, has worked with HeartBrand.

He guided a breeding program which produces 3000 full-blood cows and sells 400-500 bulls a year for HeartBrand which markets premium branded beef from about 10,000 Akaushi-blood cattle throughout the US and overseas – including in Japan before he started his own consultancy in 2016. As an acknowledged Akaushi genetics expert and head of 33 Ventures LLC, Dr Cooper continues to advise HeartBrand and cattle breeders across the US, Australia, South America and South Africa.

On his fourth visit to Australia, he was accompanied this month by HeartBrand president Jordan Beeman who has headed the American Akaushi Association – his parents Ron and Joan and HeartBrand itself are association life members and Dr Cooper is a registered full-blood breeder member.

They attended a three-day quarterly scientific retreat at the CY O'Connor Centre for Innovation in Agriculture at North Dandalup. Other guests included Larry Ludeke, also from Texas and president of the American International Charolais Association, Bruce Campbell, Cooara Charolais stud, Keysbrook and Victorian bovine embryologist Dominic Bayard, who breeds cattle as Goorambat Wagyu and who transfers and exports embryos as Global Reproduction Solutions.

Some of the discussion at the retreat related to merits of the Akaushi breed and potential benefits to local herds through introduction of Akaushi genetics. According to Dr Cooper, the Akaushi breed "is a more complete beef production animal, both from the maternal and terminal aspects", than Wagyu. Akaushi look more like traditional heavy-framed beef cattle and have a better carcase. They are fertile, produce good weight calves and as good mothers look after them with more milk than Wagyu cows produce, Dr Cooper said. They are hardy, tolerate heat, gain weight quickly and efficiently, can be finished at 18-24 months in a feedlot and produce flavoursome beef with the intense fat marbling of Wagyu and less trim fat than other breeds, he said.

Like Wagyu, Akaushi beef contains a higher concentration of monounsaturated fat relative to saturated fat – basically, more 'good' low-melting-point fat that is readily metabolised and less 'bad' fat that builds up around internal organs and can cause health problems. It is also a good source of oleic acid, the main constituent of olive oil. Medical research is showing these factors – higher caloric intake of monounsaturated fats combined with oleic acid – contribute to a low incidence of cardiovascular disease in people with Mediterranean-style diets.

Dr Cooper said importantly, Akaushi interbreed very well with Wagyu and many other breeds with their advantageous traits transferred to first and second-cross progeny. In Texas, Akaushi bulls are mainly crossed with "British-based breeds" such as Hereford, but may also be crossed with Brangus or Santa Gertrudis to improve production "efficiency" and end-product "eating quality", he said. Dr Cooper said initially Akaushi beef was marketed in the US on its healthier qualities compared to other beef. "But the marketing has changed and the better health aspect is now a sideline," he said. "The main marketing impetus is around the eating experience, the better flavour and texture of the Akaushi beef is what continues to sell the product.

"The American consumer likes a thick steak and wants to feel full and satisfied at the end of the meal. "The marbling enables that and has a consistency something like butter and a nutty flavour which they really like. "From a restaurant perspective, you can tell people Akaushi beef is the healthiest around and customers will try it. "But it has to have the flavour and the texture they expect from a premium steak otherwise they won't order it again." Dr Cooper confirmed "the Akaushi influence" was still developing in the US – Texas ranchers used a since closed loophole in trade legislation with Japan to import eight Akaushi cows and three bulls in the mid 1990s which became the foundation herd.

That foundation herd is the source of most Australian Akaushi bloodlines, but Australia is lagging a long way behind in utilising the breed's traits, he said. "In my view, Australian cattle producers are leaving a lot of money on the table by not adopting Akaushi genetics," Dr Cooper said. But that could change with an ongoing sharing of information between WA and US Akaushi breeders, shared scientific studies and a local involvement in a US-based breeding program...

John Dawkins visited Texas and HeartBrand in 2015, inspecting feedlots with up to 80,000 cattle and learning about the breed. Since then TMG's Akaushi herd has grown to the point where "we have more reds than blacks" and has superseded Wagyu as preferred commercial cross with Simmental cows, Mr Dawkins said. "In our own (TMG) program, with a full-blood red bull over Simmental females we are able to get the same weight gains and carcase weight in our first cross as we get in Simmental, but we also get the marbling as well," he said. "The trick they (Akaushi) have over the black (Wagyu) is that they can improve normal beef and fit into our short-fed program. "In our 100-day program the first crosses do extraordinarily well – you wouldn't get that with the blacks and you wouldn't get the marbling to the same extent in that time frame."

Mr Dawkins said TMG planned to set up a "small but not insignificant" breeding program in Texas in collaboration with Dr Cooper, starting with about 30 head and looking to improve the breed. First aim is to produce a Poll animal. "The plan is we can send embryos in both directions," he said.

...

Meanwhile Mr Dawkins said genetic testing and haplotypes (sections of genetic material that determine certain characteristics) testing is continuing to achieve homozygous (two copies of the same haplotype) consistency in first cross genetics.

Apart from "tremendous potential" to improve production of northern Australian cattle through infusion of Akaushi genetics, he said TMG and the CY O'Connor Centre were hoping to investigate potential improvement in dairy herds. "By identifying the right haplotype it might be possible to give dairy farmers something to sell by increasing the size of their calves," Mr Dawkins said. Within its own Akaushi expansion program, Mr Dawkins said TMG was considering a "buy-back" system similar to that offered by HeartBrand in the US where it sold bulls to breeder clients and offered to buy DNA-certified half-blood progeny for its branded beef program at market price plus a guaranteed premium.

Dr Cooper said he could foresee awareness of the Akaushi breed and its merits growing in Australia over the "next four to five years". "I see much potential for it," he said. "Whether we are talking about the northern part of the continent where you can cross them with a heavier bos Indicus or Brahman type female or whether you come down to a red-hided bos Indicus or a British based breed such as a Shorthorn, all those combinations are going to work very well. "We've seen that work exceptionally in America."

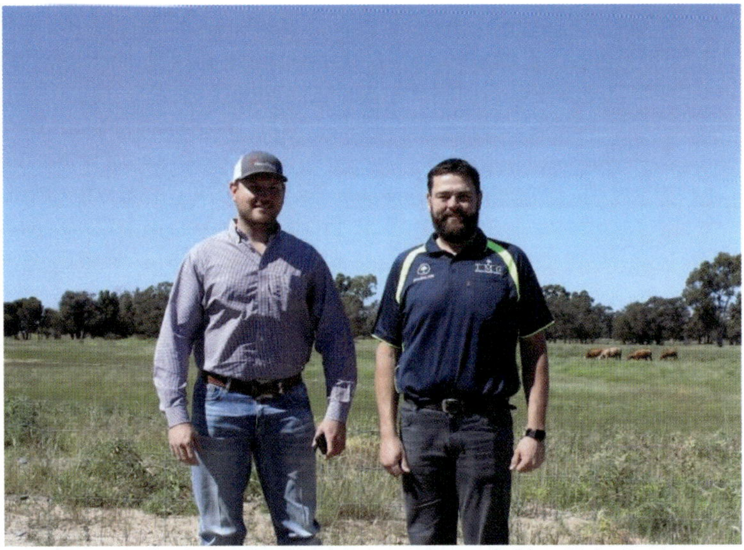

Visiting Texas authority on Akaushi cattle Aaron Cooper (left) and John Dawkins, Tillbrook Melaleuka Group, who is using Akaushi genetics to improve beef production in Simmental cattle.

Travel Reports

A WA Study Tour of Red Wagyu and Akuashi Cattle in Texas - Alan Peggs

Recently John Dawkins, CEO, Tillbrook Melaleuka Group and Alan Peggs, Deputy Chair of the C Y O'Connor ERADE Village Foundation, North Dandalup undertook a study tour in Texas to understand how – Red Wagyu - correctly known as 'Akaushi' – cattle are raised, fed, processed and marketed in Texas. In addition both John and Alan attended the American Akaushi Association's Annual Convention in Austin.

Akaushi cattle originate from the southernmost tip of the Japanese island of Kyushu. They were imported into both the United States and Australia in the mid 1990's. Like their black 'cousins' the Akaushi has an ability to produce highly marbled beef with low melting temperature fat. These attributes ensure Akaushi beef consistently eats well and improves human health by lowering cholesterol levels!

Market for Akaushi Beef

John and Alan first visited HeartBrand Beef in Flatonia, in South Central Texas. HeartBrand Beef deals exclusively in Akaushi beef. As the name suggests HeartBrand Beef focuses on the eating quality and health attributes of the Akaushi breed. Every animal which goes on feed for HeartBrand Beef is DNA tested to ensure it is at least 50% Akaushi. This ensures HeartBrand Beef can offer products which consistently eat well. Studies by HeartBrand Beef indicate it only requires one cross with Akaushi to generate the benefits of higher marbling and lower melting temperature fat.

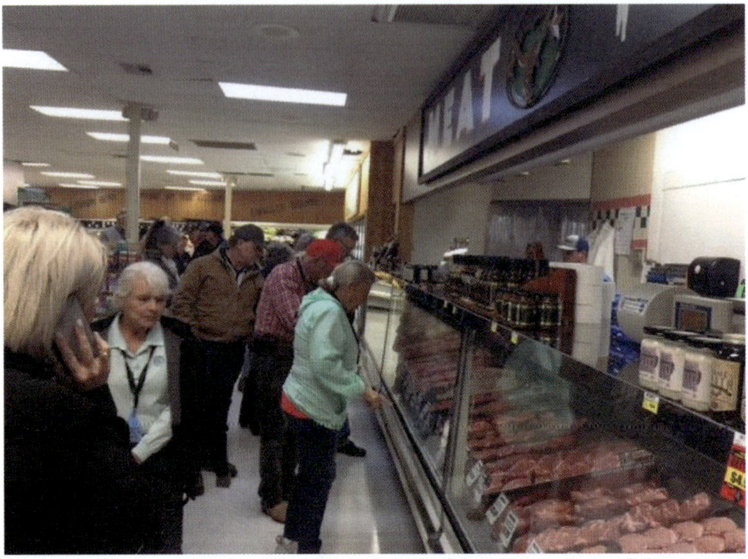

Photo 1: Delegates to the American Akaushi Association Annual Convention viewing HeartBrand Beef in the beef cabinet of a Fresh Plus store, an up-market supermarket, in Austin Texas

Currently HeartBrand Beef processes around 100,000 head annually. According to the CEO of HeartBrand Beef, Jordan Beeman, demand is so great for their beef that they could market at least twice this number if they had the cattle. It was to this end Jordan visited Western Australia and the Tillbrook Melaleuka Group last year with a view to developing an additional supply chain to service demand for HeartBrand Beef in the Middle East and South East Asia out of Western Australia. HeartBrand Beef markets their products to supermarkets, the food service sector and 'on-line'. Their on-line service can deliver 'fresh' beef within twenty four hours of an on-line order being placed. They use a special polystyrene box with dry ice to keep the product 'chilled' through-out its journey to the consumer.

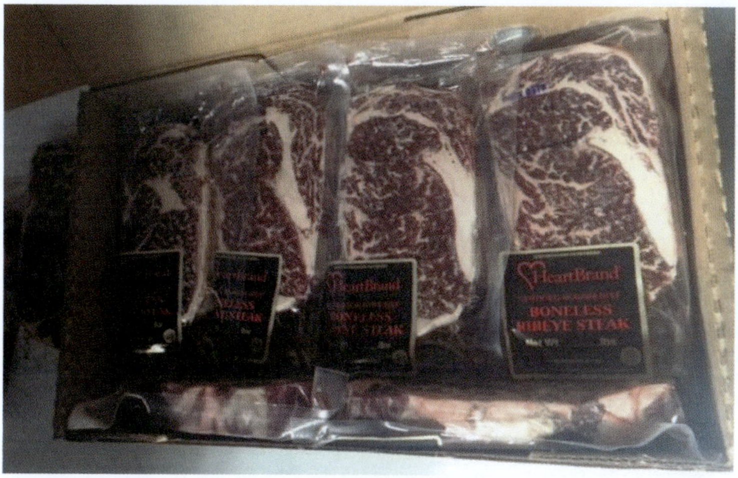

Photo 2: Highly marbled HeartBrand Rib Eye Steaks ready to be dispatched to an on-line consumer

On a ‘Taste of Akaushi Austin Style’ tour, delegates to the Annual Convention visited a ‘Taco Deli’ store where the owners explained they preferred to buy HeartBrand beef, despite it being more expensive, because they never have customers complaining about the eating quality of the beef they serve in their tacos! Taco Deli now has ten stores located in Austin, Fort Worth and Dallas. They will open a further two in Austin later this year.

Uptake of Akaushi Genetics

The American Akaushi Association celebrated its 25th Anniversary this year. Its Annual Convention held between 11th and 13th October attracted 280 delegates. While most came from the United States there were also delegations from Australia, Mexico, New Zealand and South Africa. While at the Convention delegates visited the nearby Elgin Breeding Service, an AI centre, where we saw a consignment of 30,000 straws of Akaushi semen destined for Brazil.

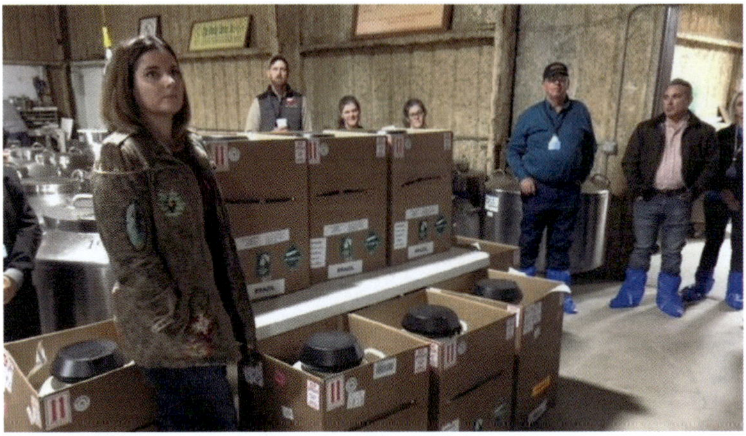

Photo 3: American Akaushi Association Annual Convention delegates visit Elgin Breeders Service, Austin, Texas to see 30,000 straws of Akaushi semen being prepared for export to Brazil.

One reason for the enthusiastic uptake of Akaushi genetics is the price premium producers receive. Jim and Corrine Yancy, who operate the 1700 ac Yancy Ranch just out of San Antonio with 200 breeding cows, said they began using Akaushi bulls over their Angus and Brangus cows because of the premium their F1 Akaushi x Angus/Brangus weaners could generate over their straight bred Angus/Brangus weaners. An F1 Akaushi x Angus/Brangus weaner at 550 lbs lw (220 kg lw) will bring US$1.60/lb (AU$5.25/kg) while a straight Angus/Brangus weaner the same weight will only bring $1.25/lb (AU$4.10/kg). It is this 28% price premium which makes it attractive to both farmers and ranchers to mate their cows to Akaushi bulls.

While the number of pedigree herds has grown to supply Akaushi bulls to commercial beef farmers and ranchers, HeartBrand Beef itself has the largest Akaushi herd in the United States – 3000 cows – spread over four ranches in South Central and South Texas.

HeartBrand Beef sells more than 300 bulls annually as well as a substantial volume of semen to cattlemen both in the United States and around the world – including Australia.

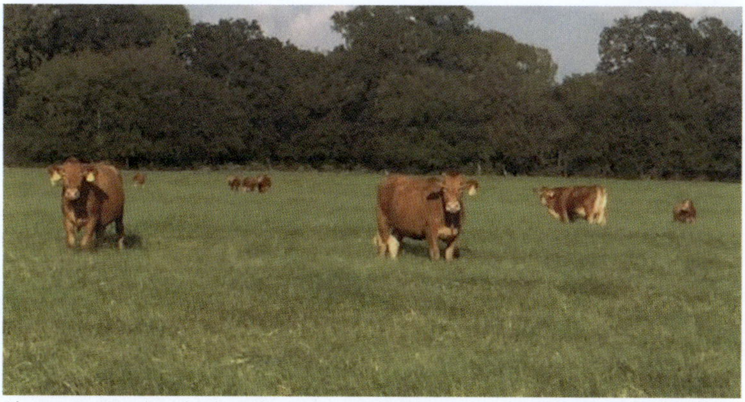

Photo 4: Purebred Akaushi cows and calves on the Beeman Ranch, Harwood, Texas grazing Bermuda grass pastures – 40 inch rainfall zone.

Ability to Perform in 'Tough' Environments

Another reason for the uptake of Akaushi genetics in the United States is their ability to thrive in 'tough' environments.

As part of John and Alan's study tour they visited two ranches in what is considered 'low' rainfall country by Texas standards.

The first was the Myers-Cooper Ranch, just south of San Angelo, in West Texas. This region normally receives 18 inches of annual rainfall but at the time of John and Alan's visit had only received 10 inches for the year. Typically the region is characterized by Mesquite trees and prickly pear cactus! The Myers-Cooper Ranch is around 2500 acres and runs 200 breeding cows – one cow to 25 acres. Most of the cows are 'stud' cows with a number being embryo recipients. Despite the harsh environment Akaushi cattle do remarkably well. The ranch is run by Dr Aaron Cooper, who is a consultant livestock geneticist specializing in the Akaushi breed. Dr Cooper has clients through-out the United States as well as Latin America, South Africa and Australia. He has visited Western Australia a number of times.

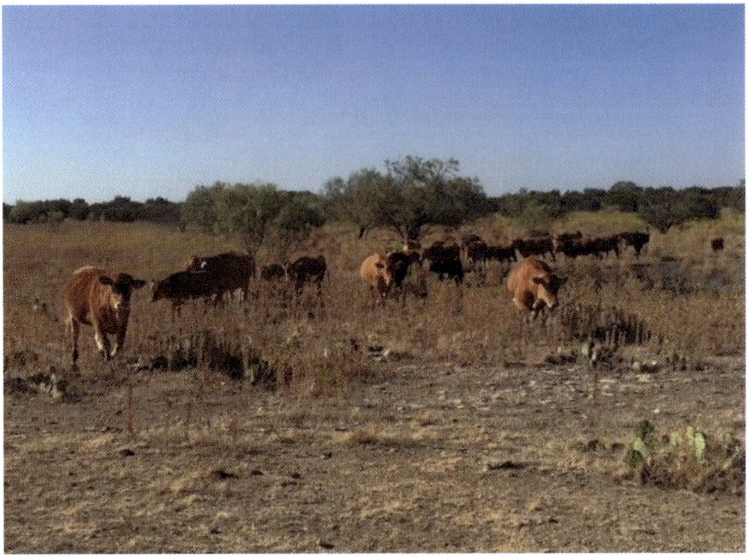

Photo 5: Purebred Akaushi cows and calves on the Myers-Cooper Ranch, San Angelo, West Texas – prickly pear cactus in the foreground and Mesquite trees in the background.

The second ranch John and Alan visited was Jim and Kelli Dyers's Rancho Espuela Ranch at Fort Davis in South West Texas– just 30 miles from the Mexican border. This ranch is in a 16 inch rainfall zone and is 5000 feet above sea-level. Unlike the Myers-Cooper Ranch it had received its annual 16 inch rainfall and as a consequence, according to Jim, John and Alan were seeing the ranch in its 'Sunday clothes'! The ranch totals 25,000 acres and normally runs one cow to 45 acres. He currently runs around 400 breeders and 130 heifers. Jim was originally a black Limousin breeder and bred his Akaushi herd up from this base. In addition he also purchased purebred females in order to produce bulls for sale to other ranchers.

Jim has one of the few heterozygous poll 15/16ths Akaushi bulls in the world. He currently markets the semen at US$100/straw. Semen will be available in Australia in the near future. 'El Padino', at the Grow Safe System bull test centre in Canyon, Texas, achieved a live weight gain of 1.92 kg/day over a 69 day test period with an average dry matter feed conversion of 5.44:1.

In addition to being a rancher, Jim is also President of the First State Bank of Fort Davis and operates a company called Big Bend Trailers which manufactures cattle trailers in Mexico for sale in the United States.

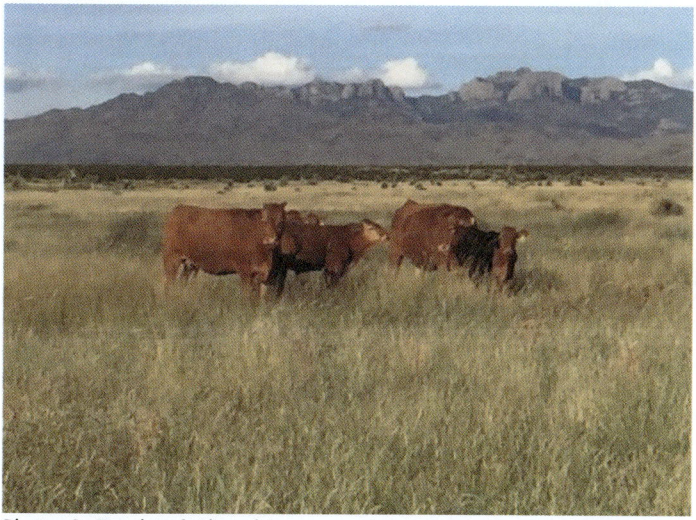

Photo 6: Purebred Akaushi cows and calves on Jim Dyer's Rancho Espuela Ranch, Fort Davis, South West Texas.

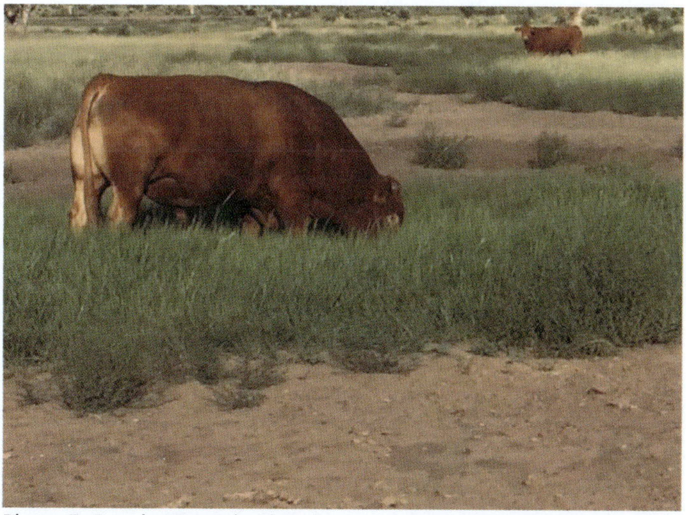

Photo 7: Rancho Espuela El Padrino – Jim Dyer's heterozygous poll $15/16^{th}$ Akaushi bull out in the 'paddock' with cows and calves on the Rancho Es-

puela Ranch, Fort Davis, South West Texas. Semen will be available in Australia in the near future.

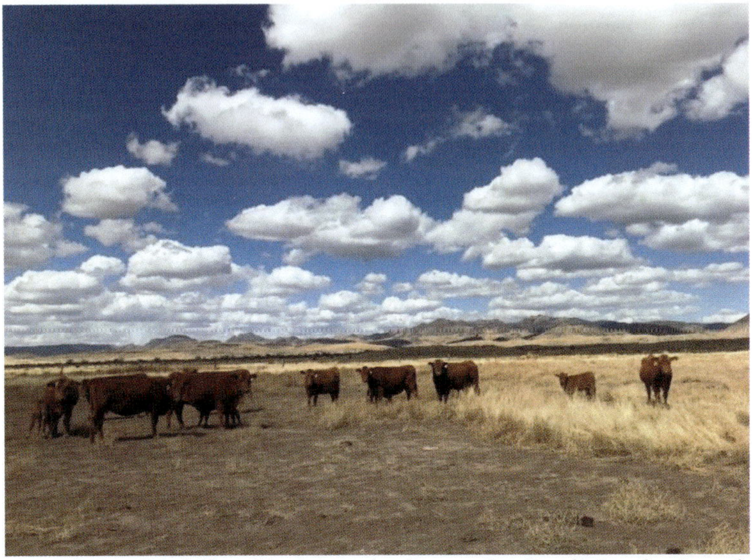

Photo 8: Purebred Akaushi cows and calves on Jim Dyer's Rancho Espuela Ranch, Fort Davis, South West Texas in a more 'normal' year!

F1 Akaushi – Best Cross-breeding Options

According to Jo Jo Carrales, Vice President, Livestock Operations, HeartBrand Beef, Akaushi cross well with a range of breeds. To date they have data on the performance of 13 F1 breed combinations with Akaushi. The HeartBrand Beef herd itself was bred up from Red Angus. Given the dominance of Angus in the United States the F1 Akaushi x Angus is the most common breed combination. However on their tour John and Alan saw a range for F1 Akaushi crosses ranging from Akaushi x Brahman to Akaushi x Jersey. All perform well in the feedlot and on the rail according to Jo Jo Carrales. Cee Arnett who is CEO, of Bovina Feeders at Farwell in the 'Panhandle' of Texas, which has a capacity to 45,000 head daily, and where HeartBrand Beef has 10,000 head fed under contract at any one time, noted there had been a substantial increase in the use of Akaushi semen in dairy herds in the Panhandle due to the easy calving attributes of the breed. Akaushi calves have an average birthweight of 30.8 kg. Bovina Feeders feed a significant number of F1 Akaushi x Holstein and F1 Akaushi x (Holstein x Jersey) steers and heifers and they perform well both in the feedlot and on the 'rail'.

John and Alan were most impressed with the F1Akaushi x Brahman heifers they saw at the HeartBrand Beef ranch. The F1 Akaushi x Brahman female would be a great female in the pastoral regions of Western Australia. The Akaushi component would dramatically improve the fertility and carcass attributes in the F1 while the Brahman component would provide environmental adaptability.

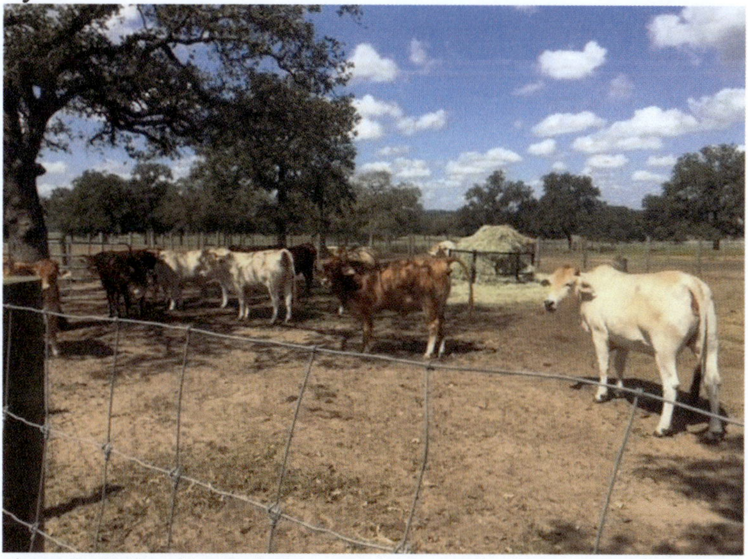

Photo 9: F1Akaushi x Brahman mated 18 month old heifers on the HeartBrand Beef Ranch, Harwood, South Central Texas.

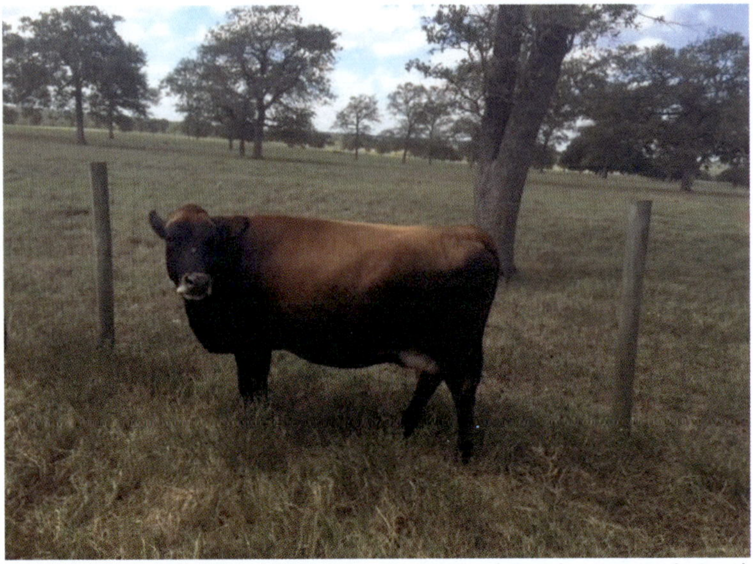

Photo 10: F1 Akaushi x Jersey HeartBrand Beef Ranch, Harwood, South Central Texas – the ranch has two Akaushi x Jersey cows to 'mother up' calves who lose their mothers at birth – which is not a regular occurrence!

Akaushi in the Feedlot and On the 'Rail'

Jim Dyer, apart from being a rancher, banker and cattle trailer manufacturer is also a pilot, which was handy as he flew John and Alan in his Cessna 210 from his ranch at Fort Davis up to Farwell in in the Panhandle of Texas – a distance of around 375 miles or 700 km. At Farwell Jim, John and Alan caught up with Cee Arnett and his team at Bovina Feeders. Here they saw some of the 10,000 Akaushi cross cattle HeartBrand Beef have on contract feed. All HeartBrand Beef animals are 'naturally' fed. This is an important distinction in the United States. It means no hormonal growth promotants or any ionophores are used in the diets of 'naturally' fed cattle. While this results in slightly slower growth rates this is a 'cost' HeartBrand Beef is prepared to 'wear' in order to ensure the health attributes of their product is maintained. (As an aside it now means they are examining the prospects of exporting beef to the European Union next year given the recent signing of the US EC Free Trade Agreement.)

Bovina Feeders steam flake all grain used in their rations. At the time of John and Alan's visit they had just switched over from corn to Hard Red Winter (HRW) wheat due to the rising price of corn relative to wheat. The Panhandle grows a significant amount of HRW wheat which is planted in September/October. In late Winter/early Spring – February-March – it is often grazed by 'stocker' cattle in order to gain weight to meet feedlot entry weight. It is then 'closed up' and left to regrow for harvest in late Spring/early Summer – May/June. In addition to wheat, feedlots in the Panhandle have access to corn, grain sorghum, corn silage, cotton seed meal and dried distillers grains (DDG).

To feed the current 43,000 head on feed Cee Arnett told John and Alan they mix one million pounds (450 t) of feed a day. They have a staff of 37 to manage, feed-out and maintain the feedlot.

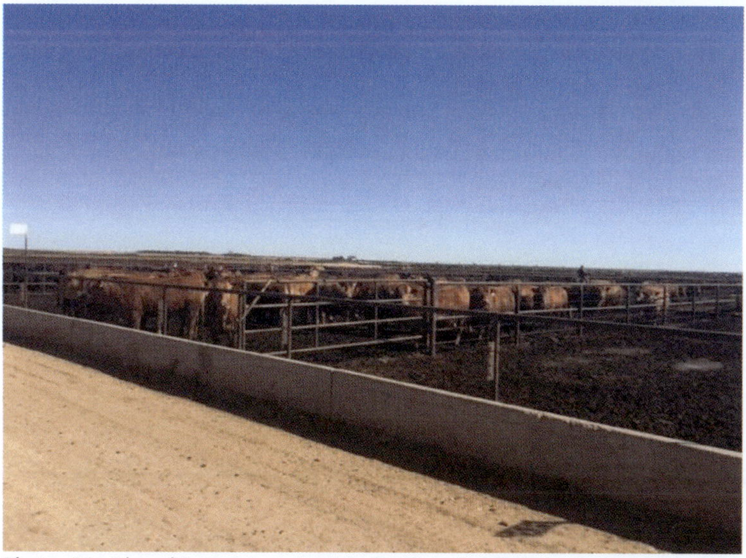

Photo 11: Akaushi steers at Bovina Feeders feedlot, Farwell, in the 'Panhandle' of Texas – despite having received 8 inches of rain the week prior to the visit by John Dawkins and Alan Peggs from Western Australia the feedlot pens were remarkably dry – a testimony to the design of the feedlot!

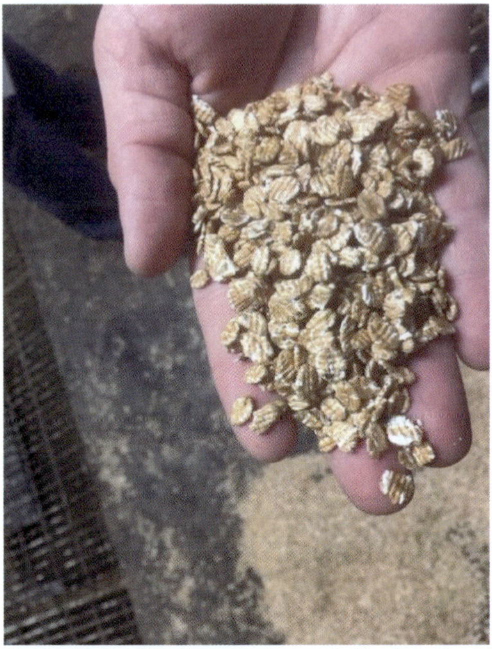

Photo 12: Bovina Feeders, Farwell, 'Panhandle, Texas steam flaked wheat – the major component of their feedlot diets.

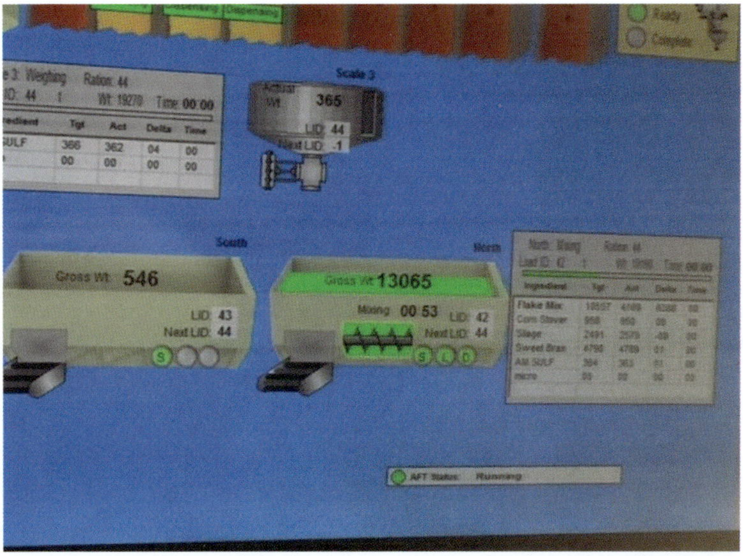

Photo 13: Computerized feed mixing at Bovina Feeders, Farwell, 'Panhandle' of Texas. The 'Flake Mix' comprises steam flaked wheat.

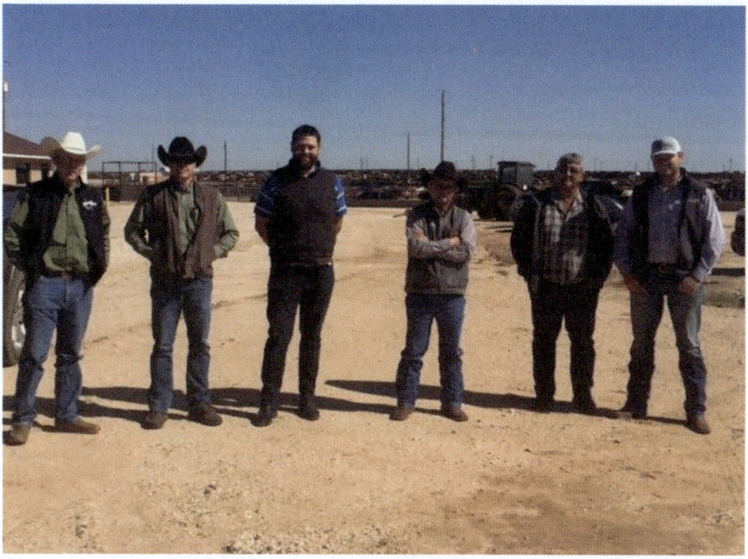

Photo 14: Bovina Feeders, Farwell, 'Panhandle' of Texas – left to right Jim Dyer, Rancho Espuela Ranch, Fort Davis South West Texas, Cee Arnett, CEO, Bovina Feeders, John Dawkins, CEO, Tillbrook Melaleuka Group, North Dandalup, WA, Darren Jones, GM, Bovina Feeders, Franz Stapelberg, President of the South African Wagyu Breeders Association and Dr Aaron Cooper, 33 Ventures, consultant livestock geneticist.

After Bovina Feeders Alan and John visited Caviness Packing Plant at Hereford just to the north of Farwell. The Caviness family have been in the beef processing sector for three generations. It is a family owned company with plants in Texas and California. At the Hereford plant they mainly slaughter and bone out cull cows and bulls for 'grinding' beef. They have a major contract to supply hamburger patties for school lunches throughout Texas. However they also provide contract slaughter and boning services. HeartBrand Beef uses Caviness packing plant to slaughter their Akaushi cattle fed at Bovina Feeders feedlot. At the time of their visit 219 steers of varying Akaushi percentage – mainly 50% and 75% - were being graded by United States Department of Agriculture graders. Unfortunately no cameras are allowed in the packing plant so no photographs could be taken by John or Alan. However of the 219 steers graded, 62% graded Prime and the remainder graded Choice. None graded Select. HeartBrand Beef expect 60% of the carcasses to grade Prime, 56% to grade Choice and 4% Select. Those carcasses which grade Select usually have a percentage of *Bos indicus* content. By way of comparison the industry average in the United States is for only 2% of carcasses to grade Prime, 53% Choice and 45% Select or No Roll. It is the marbling in the Akaushi carcasses which enables them to grade so much better than other breeds in the United States.

While at the Caviness packing plant John and Alan were accompanied by Dr Dale Woerner, Professor of Meat Science, Texas Tech University at Lubbock. Dale gave an extremely informative commentary on the merits of the carcasses being graded, the USDA grading system, the use of a highly specialized camera (made in Germany and costing US$300,000) to determine marbling levels and carcass yields in 'real' time and how different feeding regimes and grains impact on marbling and yield. After Dale's commentary both John and Alan felt they had just completed Meat Science 101 it was so comprehensive!

American Akaushi Association Annual Convention

John and Alan attended the American Akaushi Association's Annual Convention with 280 other delegates. The Convention comprised a combinations of local tours, entertainment and socializing in the evenings, a trade show with a range of exhibitors and a round of presentations focusing on 'fake' meat, lobbying by the National Cattleman's Beef Association in Washington DC to protect the beef industry from 'adverse' legislation and the importance of feeding cows appropriately in all three trimesters of gestation. John and Alan found the presentations interesting and informative. They were impressed with the quality of the presentations and the public speaking ability of the presenters.

While at the Convention both John and Alan canvassed delegates about their interest in attending an International Akaushi Convention in Western Australia next year. Many delegates, including those from Mexico, New Zealand and South Africa, indicated they would be very keen to attend such as convention. A formal proposal will be put to the American Akaushi Association to support the holding such a convention in Western Australia in October 2020 in the very near future. Tentatively the Board of the Association have said they would be in favour of such an endeavour.

In summary John and Alan considered the study tour showed:

1. there is very high demand for Akaushi beef due to its eating quality and health attributes;
2. this demand has resulted in substantial price premiums for F1 Akaushi cattle compared to straight bred cattle;
3. the Akaushi breed is very versatile – it can thrive in both 'tough' and 'benign' environments;
4. the Akaushi breed crosses very well with virtually all breeds including both *Bos indicus* and dairy; and
5. the Akaushi has great potential in the both the agricultural and pastoral regions of Western Australia.

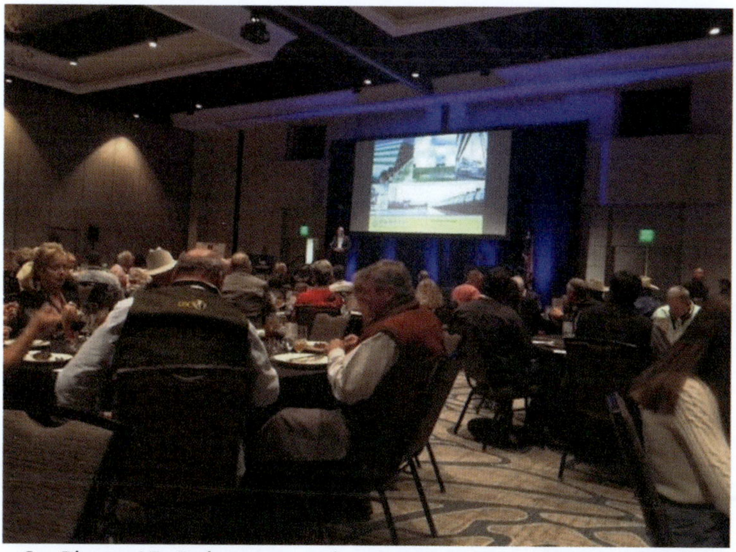

6. Photo 15: Delegates to the American Akaushi Association, Annual Convention 2019, Austin, Texas.

For more information on the Akaushi breed in Western Australia, next year's study tour to Texas in June 2020 and the International Akaushi Convention in WA October 2020 contact John Dawkins on 0428-883-310 or Alan Peggs on 0428-932-717.

Events

Weekly Research Meetings

Each Wednesday throughout the year, CY O'Connor Foundation holds a one hour research meeting to share knowledge and research opportunities. The meetings are held at the Centre for Innovation in Agriculture, North Dandalup.

- Topics discussed throughout 2018 have included:
- Beef feeding trials
- Ethics requirements
- Metabolomics of beef marbling and flavour
- Bovine Johne's Disease
- Business Incubators
- Potential of solar power in irrigation and farming systems
- Biogas generators
- Tracing provenance in foods
- Transform Peel project
- Agricultural applications of networked sensors and drones
- Facial recognition technology for cattle
- Local employment opportunities
- Characteristics of C4 grasses
- Testing for adulteration of honey
- Histology of Marbling in cattle
- DNA testing for Pasture composition
- Sugar content test for silage making

Guests (September – December)

Facial Recognition in cattle	*Geoff Trowbridge*
On farm Biogas generators	*Philipp Krahman*
Meat quality improvement in Pork	*Torben Sorensen*
Incubator Support initiatives	*Andrew Outhwaite* *Tim Inglis* *Gerard Spoelstra*
Inflammatory myopathies	*Louise Smyth*
Southern Dirt	
Agristart	*Tash Ayers*
SNP Testing	*Jason Ledger, XYTOVET*
Landcare Grants	*Paula Pownall*
Peel Harvey Catchment Soil Testing Program	*Megan Le Roy*

Drone use for weed control	*Stratus Imaging*
Managing Water in the Peel Region	*Grant Rensburg*
Water Sampling in the Peel Tributaries	*Brad Degens, DWER*
Buffelo Grass for Northern Pastures	*Ray Candy*

Feedback

"Attending the Wednesday research meetings at North Dandalup provided my team with important opportunities to share the results of our investigations into the Peel Food Zone with local farmers. We listened to locals with many combined years of experience farming in the Peel and their feedback has influenced future planning for the Peel Food Zone."

Heather Percy, Manager Peel Food Zone project

"I really enjoyed my visit today and experiencing the great atmosphere you and Roger have created. It is an enormous compliment to Roger, to build this research and education unit out there in the country at the coal face of where it is needed."

Jorg Imberger

Scientific Retreats 2018

February Program

Thursday 08th February – Saturday 10th February

Symposium 1: Water and Pastures 9:00-10:40

Chair: Tony Lloyd

Waters and Pastures — Rob Giura
Rehabilitation of Pastures — Tara Reid
Northern Pastures — Ray Candy
Irrigated Pasture Production — Michael Maclaughlin
Peel Airborne Electromagnetic Survey — Andy Ellet
'Increasing the digestibility of Kikuyu grass using new breeding technologies' — Michael Jones

Symposium 2: Theories of everything

Chair: Roger Dawkins

The theory of Innovation — Roger Dawkins
Innovation within the Peel Region — Paul Fitzpatrick
The history of Gravity — Sally Lloyd
Magnets and their uses — Roger Dawkins for Michael Maclaughlin

Symposium 3: Business Incubator Proposals

Chair: Paul Fitzpatrick

Technology needed for Car Restoration — Davyd Hooper
Satellite Lab testing for the Peel — Mark Castalenelli
Insect Farming: Closing the Production Cycle — Paula Pownall
Testing needs by MZI — Neil Graham
Has Modern Breeding made Wheat More Toxic — Chris Florides

Tour of Peel and Murdoch

Mucca Dairy Robotic Milking, North Dandalup
Green Acres Turf Farm, Nambeelup
State Agricultural Biotechnology Centre, Murdoch University

Conference Dinner Speakers

The real history of Peel — Roger Dawkins
HeartBrand, and Trends in the USA Aaron — Cooper

Friday 9th February

Symposium 4: Feeding Livestock

Chair: Sally Lloyd

Low Lignin Oats and Feed Value — Alan Peggs
Feeding Wagyu — Geoff Lister
Barley and Kikuyu BACD — Joanne Rollinson
Reducing the Allergenicity of Wheat — Mike Jones

Feeding Livestock	Dean Maugham
A2 Milk Production and Pastures	Michael MacLaughlin

Symposium 5: Strength and Weaknesses of the red meat industry

Chair: Paul Fitzpatrick

Haplotypes for Marbling	Dom Bayard
Weaknesses: Fruit and Nuts	Roger Dawkins
Strengths: Beef Industry in Japan	John Dawkins

Symposium 6: Threats of the red meat industry

Chair: John Dawkins

Bovine Johnes Disease in Victoria	Dom Bayard
Carcass Identification through Haplotyping	Jose Valenzuela
Lab Practice and Certification	Sally Lloyd
Anti-Red Meat Lobbies	Aaron Cooper

Symposium 7: Opportunities of the red meat industry

Chair: Alan Peggs

Sequencing C19 Haplotypes	John Blinco
Opportunities: Irrigated Pasture in the Pilbara	Alan Peggs
Recognition of Health Benefits	Sally Lloyd
Optimizing Volatile Fatty Acids	Roger Dawkins
Proposals for Melaleuka Red Wagyu	Aaron Cooper

Saturday 10th February: Practical sessions at Roebrooks Yards and C Y O'Connor Laboratory

Session 1: Bull Assessment **led by Aaron Cooper**
Session 2: Research and training with embryo Transfer

October Program

Thursday 11th: Centre for Innovation in Agriculture

Chair: Roger Dawkins

Current haplotyping	Sally Lloyd
Future haplotyping (SNP v Ancestral Haplotypes)	John Blinco
Marbling	Jose Valenzuela
TM	Sally Lloyd
Industry needs Australia	Dom Bayard
North America	Aaron Cooper
XYTOVET	Jason Ledger
Gyulais	Danny Hammond
Charolais	Larry Ludeke
Charolais Haplotypes	Sally Lloyd
Heart Brand	Jordan Beeman
Commercial Opportunities	Burditt Krost

Dinner Talks : "In Defence of the Cow"

Roger Dawkins, Alan Peggs, John Macaulay, Aaron Cooper, Jordan Beeman

Friday 12th: Centre for Innovation in Agriculture

Chair:John Dawkins

Silage making Demonstration	Philipp Krahmann
Rye Grass pastures and endophytes	Ray Candy
Feed trial	Jose Valenzuela
MLA Grant	Sally Lloyd
Grasses and BACD	Tony Lloyd - Joanne Rollinson
Applications of mass spectrometry to small molecule profiling	Joel Gummer
Soils for Life Project (RED Grant)	Grant van Rensburg
Problem Solving in Peel (PSIP)	Paul Fitzpatrick

Saturday 13th: Embryo Flushing Demonstration

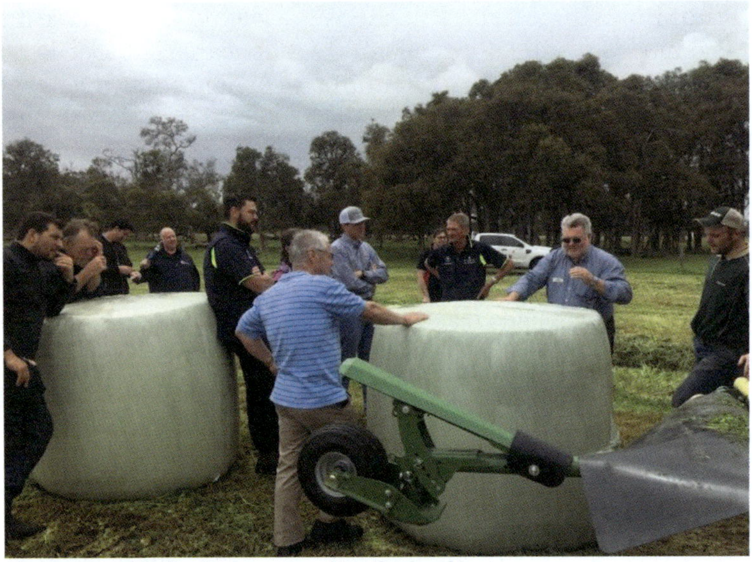

Alan Peggs and Philipp Krahmann explain silage making.

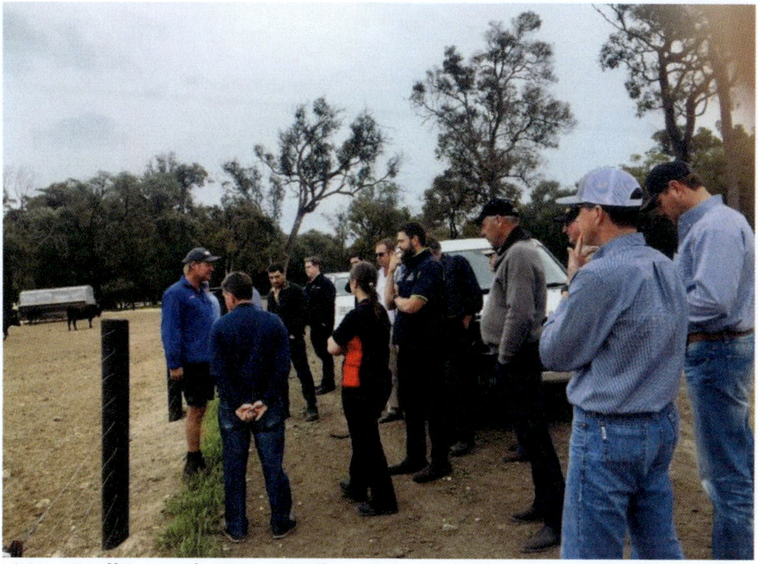

Visit to Geoff Pearson's Wagyu Feedlot

Invited Speakers:

Prof Roger L Dawkins, Chairman - CYO Foundation
Mr Tony Lloyd, Vice Chair - CYO Foundation and PSIP
Dr Sally Lloyd, Director Research Lab - CYO Foundation
Mr Paul Fitzpatrick - CYO Foundation and PSIP
Mr Jordan Beeman – HeartBrand, Texas
Mr Dom Bayard – Global Reproductive Solutions/Cutting Edge Genomics, Vic
Dr Sam Dawkins - CYO Foundation Member
Mr John R Dawkins – Tillbrook Melaleuka Group
Dr Jose Valenzuela - CYO and Melaleuka Stud
Mr Ben Dawkins - CYO Foundation Board
Mr Alan Peggs – Pastoral Consultant, WA
Mr Jim Brennan - Brennan Mayne Agribusiness, Qld
Mr John Blinco – Murdoch University
Dr Louise Smyth – Murdoch University
Mr Rob Giura – Peel Dairy Farming, PSIP and CYO Board
Dr Josh Sweeney – Milne Feeds
Dr Aaron Cooper – 33 Ventures, San Angelo, Texas, USA
Ms Paula Pownall – Grubs Up Australia
Professor Chengdao Li – Murdoch University
Mr Ray Candy – Selected Seeds
Mr Philipp Krahmann - Rosher
Mr Ric Hunter – Bald Ridge Wagyu, Texas, USA
Dr Nick Stone - Kryatec, Qld
Dr Ivan Himawan - Queensland University of Technology

Additional Guests:

Mr. Adrian Pitsikas - Greenacres Turf, Serpentine
Mr Graeme Brickwood, - Serpentine Transport
Mr Renny Lee Steere - CYO Foundation Board
Mr Wayne Cox - CYO Foundation Board
Mr Patrick Dawkins - CYO Foundation Board
Mr Bruce Campbell – Peel Livestock Farming and PSIP
Dr Hillary Nath – EcoAdvise
Mr Jeremy Allen – Jingilli Cold Pressed Olive Oil
Mr Michael McLaughlin - Jersey Milk WA
Dr H (Reb) Rebhan – PSIP
Mr Grant van Rensburg – PSIP
Mr John McCaulay – PSIP
Mr Cam Petricevich – PSIP
Mr Geoff Manning – PSIP
Mr Jim Mitchell – PSIP
Cr Brenda Beacham – PSIP
Mr Davyd Hooper – PSIP
Mr Mike Walmsley – PSIP
Mr Leigh Mclarty- Farmer, Peel Region
Mr Doug Hall – Pastoralists and Graziers Association WA
Mr Anthony Snell – Farmer, Peel Region
Mr Ric Letari – Farmer, Peel Region

* * *

December Program

Wednesday 12th

Dawkins Family Christmas Party
Launch of Australian Akaushi Branch

Thursday 13th

Symposium 1: Improving Meat Quality in Northern Beef

Market for Grass Fed Australian Akaushi in America	Aaron Cooper
Red Wagyu advantages as F1	Sally Lloyd
Bundarra Santa Gertrudis	Mel and Matt Leeds
Grazing Innovation	Greg Brennan
Improving meat quality in northern beef	Alan Peggs
Fixed wing drones and spectral imaging: capabilities for monitoring cattle	Geoff Trowbridge
Remote monitoring: needs of the pastoral industry	Doug Hall
Cattle at Mt Augustus Station	Matt Hammarquist
Continuously monitoring cattle through ear tags	LoRaWAN technology

Parallel Session: Pasture Program

Chair: Paul Fitzpatrick

Soils for Life	Terry Harkness
Soil Carbon	Simon Dawkins
Kikuyu for soil improvement	Tony Lloyd/RL Dawkins
Tour of Melaleuka Stud	

Parallel Session: Beef Program

Digital Beef, AAA registration and data collection, Q&A — Abby Hunter/Sally Lloyd
Parentage verification Sally Lloyd
Cattle Assessment (Roebrooks Yards) — Rick Hunter, JR Dawkins, L Baker

Friday 14th December

Olfactory receptors and the Multifunctional Polymorphic Controller	Roger Dawkins
Free fatty acid receptor function in ruminants	Sally Lloyd
Murdoch Metabolomics	Joel Gummer for Simon Cook
Measuring flavour compounds from grass fed beef	Joel Gummer
Consumer preference testing and flavour compounds	John Blinco
FFAR Polymorphism	Sally Lloyd

CYOEVF Project Proposals Presented to External Panel

Panel: Philipp Kemp, Andrew Outhwaite, David Beatty, Roban Clarke, John Hartley, Paul Fitzpatrick
CYOEVF Incubator Program — Roger Dawkins

Problem Solving in Peel	Paul Fitzpatrick
Biogas Generation	Philipp Krahman
Applications of FFAR haplotypes	Sally Lloyd
Facial Recognition for the cattle crush	Geoff Trowbridge
Biopsy for sequential monitoring of marbling	Jose Valenzuela
Silver stains for visualising unsaturated fatty acids	Gerard Spoelstra
Red Wagyu for the Southern Rangelands	Alan Peggs
Sequencing	John Blinco

Saturday 15th, Roebrook Yards

Cattle Assessment: Rick Hunter, B Campbell, Phil & Cam Petricevich

* * *